Health Policy a

D0539732

Other titles edited by Deborah Hennessy
Community Health Care Development (Macmillan, 1997)

Other titles edited by Peter Spurgeon
The New Face of the National Health Service (Longman, 1993)
Implementing Change in the National Health Service (Chapman & Hall, 1991)

Health Policy and Nursing

Influence, Development and Impact

Edited by

Deborah Hennessy

and

Peter Spurgeon

First published 2000 by
MACMILLAN PRESS LTD
Houndmills, Basingstoke, Hampshire RG21 6XS
and London
Companies and representatives throughout the world

ISBN 0–333–73461–0 paperback

A catalogue record for this book is available from the British Library.

This book is printed on paper suitable for recycling and made from fully managed and sustained forest sources.

10 9 8 7 6 5 4 3 2 1
09 08 07 06 05 04 03 02 01 00

Editing and origination by
Aardvark Editorial, Mendham, Suffolk

Printed in Malaysia

*To nurses worldwide who struggle relentlessly to influence
the political agenda for the 'common good'*

CONTENTS

Figures

Tables

Health policy and nursing is a fascinating but neglected topic. Policy-makers and policy analysts lacking a nursing background often fail to pay close attention to it, despite the major impact that nursing has on the quality of patient care and the sheer size of the nursing workforce. Meanwhile, most nurses are too preoccupied with the pressing demands of delivering care to spend much time thinking about it.

This book makes an important contribution to redressing the balance. I am pleased to introduce it as I was a kind of midwifery assistant at the series of seminars at the University of Birmingham that preceded its birth. Many of the seminar papers were so interesting that I asked Deborah Hennessy to edit a series of them in *Nursing Times;* these form the backbone of this book.

The lack of debate on nursing and health policy both outside and within the profession is a complex phenomenon itself worthy of analysis. Some contributory factors include an assumption that nurses are merely the pairs of hands (and feet) who implement what the policy-makers decide; an undervaluing of the contribution that nursing makes to health and illness care (concomitant with an over-valuing of medical science); there are many more factors, ranging from sexism to the career structure of civil servants and academics. Yet, apart from anything else, the sheer range and fascination of the papers gathered here makes you wonder why such a fertile and inter-esting field should lie unploughed for so long.

The authors come from a wide variety of backgrounds and disci-plines, offering many perspectives. Most write with direct experience of the crucible in which policy and practice meet, whether as current or former practitioners, health service managers, development workers or scholars. Their accounts are not dryly academic, although they do contain plenty of stimulating theory and hypothesis: as one enlight-ened nurse teacher said, 'There's nothing so practical as good theory!'

Most if not all of the authors, despite their different emphases, would probably agree with Dr Hennessy's insistence in Chapter 1 on the importance of understanding policy processes better in order to influence them. The book's main focus is the involvement of nurses in the development and implementation of policies, with the subtext that greater participation in those processes is urgently needed. Amen to that, especially at a time when so many nurses feel alienated from the culture of the health service they entered with high hopes of being able to help others and find personal satisfaction in so doing. With four out of every five Trusts now reporting difficulties in recruiting nursing staff, the need to involve nurses at all levels of planning and decision-making is more pressing than ever: otherwise, solutions to the nursing crisis will remain elusive.

Furthermore, changes in the nurse's role, the shifting boundaries with medicine that are giving nurses increasing independence and authority, and changing expectations on the part of society itself all urge greater nursing involvement. Broader social change, especially in the role of women but also in the growth of stakeholder power, points the same way, trends that are reinforced by the policies of the UK Labour government elected in May 1998.

Increasingly, however, it is not just national, but also international, policies and practices that count. This book's pleasingly cosmopolitan flavour reflects that, with contributions on nursing and health policy in Australia, Canada, Central and Eastern Europe, the European Union, the USA and elsewhere. These accounts encourage transnational comparisons that provide a great stimulus to learning and discussion.

Finally, and thankfully, the contributors do not make the mistake of assuming that what policy-makers decree is what happens in real life – although, as Walsh and Gough point out in Chapter 13, poorly formulated policy can have a negative impact on practice. Spurgeon argues in Chapter 12 that policy-making is an incremental, messy process, while Hicks (Chapter 11) and Fry (Chapter 14) explore the complexity of the relationship between policy and practice.

One starting point for us, as nurses who want to influence policy, is to put our own house in order. We readily deplore the lack of notice that others seem to take of us, while also hoping that it is gradually changing – but it is dangerous to throw stones in a glass house. Much remains to be done in improving nursing's own track record of policy development. We need better policy-making processes within the profession, based on openness, genuine efforts to maximise participation, greater maturity in accepting difference and seeing it as the basis of consensus rather than something to be feared, and an ability to let go of territorial fears and personal insecurities. Such innovating and courageous processes would help us practise our fledgling policy-making skills and even provide some examples to others of how it should be done.

JANE SALVAGE, RGN, BA, MSc, HONLLD,
Editor-in-Chief, *Nursing Times*

All health personnel who are in a position to influence nursing policy and its relationship with health policy will want to read this book. It arises out of two national conferences exploring the interaction of nurses with the development of health policy. The text of the book emerges from the papers delivered at the second seminar in January 1997. Seventeen speakers, who came from the UK, Europe, the USA, Canada and Australia, were asked to prepare a 5000 word paper in advance of the seminar, covering their own specialist subject area. The authors are each known nationally, and in most cases internationally, for their contribution to health policy and nursing policy processes.

The authors were asked to link their papers to the aims of the conference, as follows. First, they were asked to continue developing confidence in identifying the critical issues for the contribution of nursing to policy development. Second, their brief was to explore the developments of related influencing strategies. Third, they were to assess whether nursing is excluded from or missing opportunities for policy involvement. Related to the last point is the identification of cohesion or competition within the nursing profession in these matters, together with demonstrations that opportunities for this work are being created or stifled.

The papers were sent to a discussant who read and prepared a critique for the seminar. The papers were not read at the seminar, instead, each of the participants had a copy of most of the papers. The discussant and the author explored the author's paper together in front of the audience. Then the audience were invited to participate. Following the discussions, the authors of the papers were invited to review and redraft their papers as chapters for this book. Both the editors of the book also prepared papers.

The rationale for writing this book is that nursing develops in response to changing social needs. The work adapts to the changes in the patterns of society and the varying demands by patients, their families and the wider public for health care provision. These changes are continuous and accelerate with the accumulation of knowledge (Baly, 1973). As we move into the next century, these changes are very rapid, dramatic and are transforming society. New styles of institution, strategic decision-making, places where work is done and the methods used are rapidly replacing those known, even in the last decade. This book is set against this background of rapid worldwide change in all organisations, managerial systems and processes. This is perhaps especially, but not exclusively, so in the West.

The changes are reflected by governments reviewing their health care systems and the suitability of their existing approach to financing, organising and delivering health care services. Health care reform is, however, an activity that is normative (reviewing and resetting standards) as well as including the examination of the financial and organisational structures. Pressures to achieve better expenditure and control have to be balanced against the deeply rooted moral imperatives to maintain universal access to essential health care. This of course implies equity in distribution geographically and across social divides. These activities need to be judged not only on short-term savings to public budgets, but also by their ability to promote health and generate health gain for entire populations (WHO Regional Office for Europe, 1966). What then, at this time in history, is the role of nursing in the development and implementation of these normative, financial and organisational health policies? Are nurses involved in the development of these policies? Do nurses understand how to use the political and economic processes so that their extensive first-hand knowledge of patients, and their needs, is reflected in policy developments? Are nurses adequately involved in the management of change that goes with implementing health policy? Do nurses speak out in appropriate forums to bring to the attention of the policy-makers the gaps in health policy that affect the quality of patient care?

The power shifts that accompany the above changes have meant that all professionals have found that their roles, work and traditional influencing processes have been challenged, and for nursing this is especially so. Nursing has fought long and hard in an unequal and perhaps unjust competition to have its experience, knowledge and wisdom acknowledged and used in the policy processes. No sooner had nurses developed their education and skills in the policy arena than the political and economical climate changed, as discussed above. The current emphasis on cost-effective, evidence-based care is placing new, and more unequal, demands on nursing to demonstrate the added value of caring for people to purchasers and providers. These demands are unequal because the structural mechanisms for enabling nurses to demonstrate that their work is cost-effective are simply not adequate. One example is the lack of user-friendly nursing management information systems.

All these challenges require fresh and interesting new approaches to facilitate the engagement of nursing with the policy processes. The purpose of this book is to explore what is happening. What approaches are nurses taking to address the current situation, and how are they getting involved in the policy processes?

REFERENCES

Baly, M. (1973) *Nursing and Social Change*. London: Heinemann.
WHO Regional Office for Europe (1996) *European Health Care Reforms: Analysis of Current Strategies*. Copenhagen: WHO.

DEBORAH HENNESSEY, BA, PhD, RN, RM,
RHV, DIP PUBLIC HEALTH NURSING

We would like to thank all those nurses and others who encouraged us to prepare this book.

A very special note of thanks to Sabrina Begum who patiently followed up the chapter authors all over the globe and lent her own special expertise to pulling the different drafts together.

Richenda Milton-Thompson of the publishers deserves a special mention for ensuring that the idea became a reality.

The editors and publisher wish to thank the *Canadian Journal of Nursing Administration* for permission to reprint all or part of the following article: Murphy, Norma J (1993) Nurses influence policy change in nursing education, *Canadian Journal of Nursing Administration*, **6**(4): 5–10.

Every effort has been made to trace all the copyright holders but if any have been inadvertently overlooked the publishers will be pleased to make the necessary arrangements at the first opportunity.

Deborah Hennessy

BA, PhD, RN, RM, RHV, Dip Public Health Nursing

Deborah has extensive experience in strategic and operational management in the UK National Health Service at a very senior level, including being Chief Nurse at St George's Hospital, London and Chief Nurse with South West Thames Regional Health Authority. She also has many years of teaching experience, especially contributing to many postgraduate degree courses related to nursing and health policy. Deborah has undertaken numerous senior management development and consultancy projects in the UK and internationally, including the USA, the Middle East, Korea, Australia, Lesotho, South Africa, Swaziland, Namibia and Zimbabwe. She has authored many publications in academic journals and a number of book chapters, and is the editor of *Community Health Care Development*, published in 1997

Peter Spurgeon

BSocSci, PhD

Peter has worked in a number of different sectors but has, for the past 15 years, been in the university and health sector arena. He is an experienced health service researcher collaborating with a number of professional groups (doctors, nurses and midwives) in research and consultancy projects. He has written and published widely in relation to health service reform, including international work (Australia, Hong Kong and Zimbabwe). Peter is editor of *Health Services Management Research* and a member of the Board of Evidence-Based Health Policy and Management

Christopher Birt

Senior Lecturer in Public Health, Health Services Management Centre, University of Birmingham

Ainna Fawcett-Henesy

BA, RN, RHV
Regional Nurse Adviser to the World Health Organisation, Geneva

Sylvia Fry
RN, RHV, DMS

Executive Director, Nursing/General Manager Locality Services Division, Southern Birmingham Community Health NHS Trust

Pippa Gough
MSc, RN, RM, RHV, PGCEA

Director of Nursing Policy Unit, Royal College of Nursing, London

Carolyn Hicks
BA, MA, PhD, CPsychol

Reader in Health Care Psychology at the School of Continuing Studies, University of Birmingham

Carole P. Jennings
PhD, RN

Professor in Health Policy and Informatics, University of Maryland, Baltimore, USA

Nora Kearney
RN

Macmillan Lecturer in Cancer Nursing, Department of Nursing Studies, University of Glasgow; President of the European Oncology Nursing Society

Tom Keighley
RN, RM, NDN Cert, DN (London), BA (Hons)

Director of International Development, School of Healthcare Studies, University of Leeds

Sandra Legg
RN, RM, BA (Hons), MSc, ThL, Dip Clin Counselling, FRCNA, FCN (NSW)

Director of Nursing, Cabrini Hospital, Melbourne, Australia; prior to this, Chief Nurse of St George's Healthcare NHS Trust, London

Norma Murphy
MSN, RN

Assistant Professor at the School of Nursing, Dalhousie University, Halifax, Nova Scotia, Canada

Kathy Redmond
MSc, RGN
Lecturer in Cancer Nursing, University College, Dublin

Trevor J. Ride
RN
Consultant in Nursing and Health Policy; Visiting Lecturer Nuffield Institute for Health, University of Leeds

Elizabeth Scott
PhD, MA, RN
Independent Consultant

Nicola Walsh
RN, MSc
Research Fellow at the Health Services Management Centre, University of Birmingham

Sonia Zyntek
MEd, BAppSc Nursing, RN, RM
Nursing Staff Development Officer, Cabrini Hospital, Melbourne, Australia

CHAPTER ONE

The emerging themes

Deborah Hennessy

In the evening you say, 'It will be fine, there's a red sky', and in the morning, 'Stormy weather today; the sky is red and overcast'. You know how to read the face of the sky, but you cannot read the signs of the times. (Matthew, 16: 3)

INTRODUCTION

The shape of nursing is determined by health policy. The text in this book explores nurses' involvement in the policy process. Nurses participate in the process sometimes at the policy development or implementation stage but most often through the impact of policy decisions on their practice. Nurses know, recognise and meet patients' immediate health and nursing care needs. However, their patients' lives and their ability to be healthy are influenced by numerous policies affecting the environment within which they live, their lifestyles, public health needs and the health services available, as well as the nursing care provided. Surely, then, nurses should know what is happening in health policy. Perhaps, in addition, it could be expected that the views of nurses, at all levels of health systems, would always be included in the development of health policy. Evidence demonstrates that nurses' views are at times sought and given, but this quite often does not happen. Percival (1997, p. 3) emphasised this: 'There are many policy roles for nurses. They drive, they navigate, they repair faults, they lubricate the engine, but they do not often design new engines.'

In this book, key nurses and others use their experiences to explore the position of nurses in policy work and how they are engaged with the health policy processes at the end of the 20th century. The different chapter authors describe situations in a number of countries, noting particularly the roles that nurses have had in influencing health policy.

The impact of health policy on nursing and nurses is frequently written about in books and in the contemporary nursing press. Therefore the content of this book focuses especially on those areas of nurses' work with policy that receive less attention, namely the involvement of nurses in the development and implementation of policies. The reason for this focus is that participation by nurses in this work is particularly urgent with the emergence of new societal values, a wider perspective of health care and different decision-making processes at government level and throughout society. These changes include nurses becoming more accountable for their actions and sharing more of the responsibility for the cost, quality and effectiveness of health care.

The present author believes that nurses have an obligation to be:

> fully involved in the policy processes, that is, in influencing the development of policies in health and other areas of community living that impinge on health, such as education, housing, child care services, employment and income distribution. There are few areas that are inappropriate for nurses to attempt to influence. (Hennessy and Swain, 1997b, p. 254)

This includes the management of the environment and ecology.

Nurses' knowledge and experiences of patients and their needs can make an essential contribution to the development of policies that are sound, just and for the common good. Appropriate ways, therefore, must be found in contemporary society for this to happen. To what degree nurses currently influence health policy is unknown. There is, however, a general belief that there could be a better recognition by nurses themselves of the opportunities and responsibility to become involved, and that they could employ more skilled influencing techniques. The rapid changes occurring as a result of health reform worldwide provide an urgency for reflection on how nurses have historically influenced policy, the current position and the way in which the nursing influence on policy processes should develop.

Although a formal course in health and social policy would be helpful in providing insight into the signs of the times, this is, for economic reasons, obviously not possible for many. A greater understanding of policy processes, as well as their history and some of the policy networks, links and power bases, would, however, make it much easier to manage the processes of influence. There is a thirst for this type of knowledge among nurses in leadership positions. If nurses better understand the history and depth of the health policy processes, they are more likely to breathe life and vigour into the power of nursing to contribute to the processes so that nursing can influence policies for the benefit of the public.

This chapter covers a number of important areas for consideration in the development of policy. Despite this, the text is not a comprehensive substitute for a textbook on the health policy process. Instead, it serves to introduce the subsequent chapters, which discuss the involvement of nurses in policy work at different health service levels. As policy development is neither a clear nor a logical process, there is an inevitable duplication of information between various chapters.

WHAT IS HEALTH POLICY?

Before discussing health policy, the concepts of health, care, nursing and nursing care, health care and policy need to be briefly discussed.

Health

A clear unambiguous definition of health is rather elusive. For many, health means an absence of disease, which implies a physiological and clinical status. Using this first definition, an abnormality in physiological functioning could imply disease.

Mulhall (1996) noted, in a second definition, that in some circumstances, abnormal physiological processes might be identified with an absence of any discernible form of disease. She also suggested that disease or physiological status does not fully comprise the image of health that most people hold. Other factors – social, physical and spiritual – are all involved in perceptions of health. In this second definition, a state of balance or harmony between the emotional, physical, social, mental and spiritual aspects of one's life could imply health. Even at the best of times, this state of health is difficult to maintain. For some individuals, families and communities, environmental factors and policies compromise the balance and put health in jeopardy.

It is important to stress that health care and health services alone cannot enable people to achieve their optimum health status (Hennessy and Swain, 1997a, p. 6). Benzeval *et al.* (1995) noted a causal link running from deprivation to poor schooling, unemployment, low earnings and poor health. The Western world's view of health, which has been equated with a narrow concern for the physical health of individuals, medical technology and its application in institutions, may prevent the population recognising many elements of health care, for example complementary medicine and environmental, cultural and spiritual factors. To illustrate this, Barker (1996, p. 13) uses the example of a malnourished peasant from a developing country:

> The doctor might wish to offer the peasant vitamins or more comprehensive nutritional rehabilitation. Were we to ask the peasant, he might argue that because his health and that for his whole family are dependent on the ox that draws the tractor he would prefer to give priority treatment to the ox.

This implies that the peasant clearly understands the relationship between the environment, health, health care and the ecosystem.

In summary, health is not only an absence of disease, but also an interrelated set of circumstances, both internal and external to an individual, that leads to one or other perceived state of health.

Care

> Care is about having concern for others; an appropriate regard; a preparedness to act; and sometimes properly, not to act. Care too, has to do with the balance, which assists in promoting independence and appropriate protection of the vulnerable from exploitation and abuse. Care and concern for others have their rightful place in the human condition in the development of the psyche. (Hennessy and Swain, 1997a, p. 8)

> The development of a capacity for concern has its roots in infancy and depends on a facilitating environment for assisting towards its eventual maturation. (Winnicot, 1990 quoted in Hennessy and Swain, 1997a).

This begins with the care and protective environment that a mother provides for her baby. The baby will not thrive without love, protection and food. Care organised via the state, voluntary services or social networks also has its benefits for the psyche. There is evidence to suggest that an altruistic approach contributes to the positive health status of individuals (Hennessy and Swain, 1997a).

Caring, Davies (1995) has said, is a fusion of labour and love that is diffuse and hard to capture, define or measure by the means known to the academic disciplines of psychology and social policy. Caring can mean just being there for someone – not necessarily even being physically present but being known to be available. 'Caring in its broadest sense can be defined as attending, physically, mentally and emotionally to the needs of another and giving a commitment to the nurturance, growth and healing of that other' (Davies, 1995, p. 140).

It is this business of attending to another, the close observation that a carer undertakes, that attunes her or him to the minute differences which are not necessarily available to the more casual or sporadic behaviour. In the public world of paid health care, the nurse is often, although not always, structurally placed to achieve this, whereas the doctor is rarely so placed. (Davies, 1995, p. 141).

Nursing care

Donahue (1996), in her book *Nursing: The Finest Art*, explores the origins of nursing, starting with the mother's care of the infant. The word 'nurse' comes from the Latin word *nutrire*, to nourish, or suckle. Over time, the meaning of the word moved on from mothering and came to include the care of young children, then spreading to a concern for all humanity. The role next expanded to include waiting on the sick, and in the last century, also to carrying out the physician's instructions. In its fullest development, nursing is altruistic and humanitarian, and has existed as a form of community service for many centuries. This is especially so as, over time, the nursing care of the sick has expanded to include concern for social problems, poverty and disease prevention, and an involvement in the social movements of the 18th, 19th and early 20th centuries. Nursing has thus been involved in public health policy for a very long time.

The concept of caring described by Davies (1995) above is complemented by the work of Parker and Wiltshire (1997, pp. 151–69), who noted that the knowledge or heart of nursing practice was rarely documented by nurses in a patient's notes. Instead, what was written was a weak record of what had already been said, usually by doctors. In order to investigate what nurses really thought, Parker and Wiltshire observed nurses' behaviour during the 'shift handover' (the time when some nurses complete their duties and hand the nursing care of their patients on to other nurses who are just beginning their shifts of patient care). Three modes of nursing practice were observed during the handover:

- The *nursing scan* is the observation and inspection of the environment around the patient, which produces local, situational and perspectival knowledge of the terrain in which the nursing takes place.
- The *nursing gaze* is similar to the medical gaze described below in the section on the power and values of health care. The gaze is the objective knowledge of the patient's body and medical history, and

includes knowledge of disease and the associated medical and nursing interventions.

● The *nursing look* conveys information that is personal to the speaker. It is the knowledge that he or she has gathered by 'being with' the patient and is a form of knowledge central to nursing care. It is seldom mentioned and hardly valued by nurses themselves.

Nevertheless when these three modes are pointed out to nurses, they always identify with them and often only then seem to recognise the depth of knowledge that they have collected in this way over time. With reflection, the three modes of nursing knowledge can be integrated and become 'a form of embodied, situated and objective knowledge'. The latter could be very powerful if complemented with data in the policy process.

Definitions of health policy

An exploration of the meaning of *policy* shows that the word may derive from the Greek *polis*, referring to a city (Sykes, 1983), whereas *politics* is the science and art of government, political affairs or life and is probably derived from the Greek word *politikos*, from *polites* a citizen or *politicus* which is Latin for political. With the passage of time, policy has acquired a number of meanings, three of which are as follows. First, a late Middle English derivation defines policy as 'a course of action adopted and pursued by a government party, ruler, statesman, etceteras; or any course of action adopted as advantageous or expedient' (*Shorter Oxford English Dictionary*, 1933). A second interpretation of policy is 'a prudent, expedient or advantageous procedure, or political course of action'. 'A crafty device, strategem or trick' is a third meaning (*Shorter Oxford English Dictionary*, 1933).

It would seem that the term 'policy' is actually very difficult to explain and tends to be defined by those who wish to study it or because something becomes an issue or a problem. (Policies are frequently neither conceived consciously nor logically developed.) Andersen (1984, p. 8) defines a policy as 'a purposive course of action followed by an actor or set of actors in dealing with a problem or matter of concern'. Health policies may therefore be described as the strategies and courses of action adopted as being advantageous and expedient to provide within the resources available from a health system that at least maintains, and preferably improves, health. In addition, the reality is that competing theories and views have to be considered. If one of these is chosen, there is a tendency to supplement it with judgement based on experience, expertise and indeed intuition (Moore, 1992).

The power and values of health care

Perhaps humans, even long before there were any known hopes of cure, have always attempted to improve the condition of their own existence and that of their communities, including by showing compassion and caring for the sick. Therefore, health care has never been the sole prerogative of medically trained personnel. This can be claimed today too, even when concentrating on only the physical aspects of health. For example, the Ministry of Transport and the police both try to reduce the incidence of trauma and the subsequent need for health care caused by motor car accidents. In society, the value of health care varies from individual to individual and society to society, as do attitudes to health (see above). For some people, health care is a fundamental right and for others a political arena that is used to secure votes by, for example, building a new hospital for which the local politician takes credit. Many governments see health care as an expenditure that must be curbed; others view it as a great investment in the development of people.

Health care is sometimes valued not for improving health but as a route to power: control over health care produces power. Governments and health purchasers hold political power over how resources will be distributed, which can lead to major political struggles. In addition, those who control the actual provision of health care wield power over individual patients (Barker, 1996).

The most powerful caring profession is undoubtedly medicine. The pre-eminent position of medicine in modern society has been very well documented, Harrison and Pollitt's (1994) work being only one example. Foucault (1973), for example, describes the emergence of 20th-century clinical medicine as the advent of a new type of clinical 'gaze' or regard that 'sees' the disease below the visible surface of the human body. We are 'dazzled by science' and forget that the genuine medical power links the knowledge of disease with the healing forces already present in individuals, their social group and the community.

Campbell (1984, pp. 18–19) refers to the views on medical power of both Talcott Parsons and Friedson. The former suggested that the service provided by doctors is socially valuable, leading to a legitimisation of their authority. Friedson, however, believed that medical dominance was a successful political move with considerable rewards in terms of dominance and power. He also thought that the greatest achievement of medical practitioners has been to persuade governments that they must be granted an exceptionally high degree of autonomy and 'ethicality'. Campbell himself expected that the position of the medical profession would probably always remain a socially dominant one. He questions whether doctors can fully use their knowledge to promote health and prevent illness as this could entail an attack on their own security.

The power of doctors is well known in health circles in many parts of the world. It is particularly important to recognise this in the UK as not only have doctors gained very high respect from society, but there is also a tradition that government civil servants, when developing health policy, will network with doctors over and above any other member of the health service. There is, however, some evidence that, over the past 10 years, general managers are also gaining considerable respect. The position of nurses is not and has probably never been comparable, although there have been one or two outstanding nurses who have been held in very high esteem, the best-known example being Florence Nightingale.

Policy decision-making

The development of a policy at any level follows decisions being taken. Andersen (1984, p. 10) describes three distinct theories of decision-making used in policy work, rational-comprehensive, incremental and mixed-scanning.

The first, *rational-comprehensive theory*, is the best known and comprises six elements:

1. There is a given problem that can be separated from other problems
2. The decision-maker has clear goals and objectives to guide his decision-making
3. The various alternatives for handling the problem are examined
4. The consequences or the costs and benefits are investigated
5. Each alternative and its consequences are examined against other alternatives
6. The decision-maker chooses the alternative that most matches his goals and objectives.

This first theory has received fierce criticism because many believe that the decision-maker seldom has a clear untangled problem or adequate information. It is also believed that the decision-maker is usually confronted with value conflicts, for example his own values compared with those of the public. Finally, there is the problem of 'sunk costs', in which a previous decision is too difficult to undo and compromises a later more rational decision. For example, a hospital once built cannot easily be shut even though there may be little need for inpatient services.

The second theory, the *incremental theory*, is said to be the more accurate description of how decisions are really made. This process usually happens in the following way (Grant, 1989):

- Goals, objectives, problems and information are intertwined and difficult to separate
- Only some of the alternatives are considered, and these will differ only marginally from existing policies
- For each alternative, only a limited number of consequences are evaluated
- The problem is continually redefined to try to make it more manageable; there is no single right decision
- The decision is usually an adjustment of current problems rather than the promotion of futuristic thinking.

Lindblom (1968) believed that this was the way in which decision-making took place in the US. It is probably also the best description of how decisions are made in the UK.

Mixed-scanning theory:

- incorporates both the earlier theories
- enables decision-makers to choose the best approach for the situation
- can be described as a sort of compromise.

Many other external factors impinge on the decision-makers, including the political values prevalent at the time, the values of the organisation, the personal values of the decision-maker and the ideological values of society. Understanding how policy decisions might be taken can be enlightening and liberating: it may help one to engage in the policy process more proactively or at least be prepared for the probable policy impact.

Policy analysis

Just as there are theories about the way in which decisions are made in policy development, there are also theories about how policy is analysed. Three of these will be discussed: the political system, group theories and élite theories (Andersen, 1984). First, the *political system theory* is one in which:

- public policy can be understood as a response to the demands of the public by the political system.

According to the second type, *group theory*:

- public policy reflects the group struggle in society
- groups juggle with each other in order to be noticed and listened to by the policy-makers
- individuals involved in policy development have to be part of an interest group or pressure group to gain any power or influence and be heard by the policy-makers
- the policy-makers referee the group struggle, and the laws and statutes demonstrate the victories.

The third type, the *élite theory*:

- has a perspective that public policy reflects the values and preferences of the governing élite and sometimes dominant groups and key figures in society
- also focuses the mind on who actually has the power in policy formulation.

In many countries, medical groups and the medical lobby are so dominant and have so much influence over health policy that they could be considered to fall into both the group and élite theories.

Nursing policy

As already stated, nurses are always involved in health policy in their day-to-day activities. Percival outlined three perspectives of nursing policy (1997, p. 7). First, nursing policy as a *philosophical concept*:

> This view sees nursing policy as a set of general principles – or a series of desirable states. Often the principles are articulated in abstract terms

but there is a search for enduring solutions to identified problems. The sort of philosophical issues at the forefront are a commitment to *quality...* equity and the recognition of rights.

The second perspective views nursing policy as a *product*. The product may be a series of conclusions or recommendations for specific or social improvement. Procedures and practice frequently back these up. The outcome could be an improvement in quality.

The third perspective is to view nursing policy as a *process* whereby organisations attempt to do and implement what is required of them. The focus is on the programmes, procedures and mechanisms for the attainment of the product, which is in turn based on the philosophical concept.

The statutory body the United Kingdom Central Council for Nursing, Midwifery and Health Visiting (UKCC) and the Nursing Boards for England, Wales, Scotland and Northern Ireland, together with the Nursing Division of the Department of Health (DoH), contribute to the development of policies and guidelines that promote standards of nursing care. Within this framework, each body has specific responsibilities to develop policies enabling nursing to meet the objectives of the overall health service, as well as to ensure that the public are protected from negligent behaviour. The nursing professional organisations in most countries contribute to the development of policies and guidelines, which support nurses in their work.

Policy formulation

The whole series of practices, statements, regulations and even laws that outline how we do things that are covered by the concept of policy do not just appear: they require proactive strategists, and there are a number of stages that may be covered during their formulation. The development and implementation of a public policy can be demonstrated by referring to the stages of the development and implementation of an Act of Parliament in the UK. The stages (using the rational-comprehensive decision-making model) are identified by Parsons (1955) thus:

1. An issue is raised
2. Networks collect information and lobby politicians and stakeholders
3. The issue may appear in a government party political manifesto or policy agenda
4. Proposals may appear in the Queen's speech

5. Green and White Papers are produced
6. Parliamentary debates take place using evidence and exploring alternatives
7. A parliamentary Bill is published, with subsequent readings and amendments in both Houses, and is followed by the Act
8. The next step is the implementation of the Act
9. Regulations appear after the publication of the Bill and the Approval of the Act
10. These are followed by circulars and codes and instructions
11. Pilot studies, detailed notes and evaluations and accounts of changing working practices appear
12. Benchmarking may be encouraged. (A benchmark is a prototype or a model of a standard that can be measured and used as a signpost. Other models can then be measured and compared with the prototype to identify the distance from the signpost.)

The above description:

> is useful for some purposes but tends to view policy-making as though it were the product of one governing mind which is clearly not the case. It fails to evoke or suggest the distinctively political aspects of policy-making, its apparent disorder and the consequent strikingly different ways in which policies emerge. (Lindblom, 1968, p. 4)

Andersen (1984) has noted three aspects of policy formation following the identification of a public problem:

- how problems come to the attention of policy-makers
- how policy proposals are formulated to deal with particular problems
- how a specific proposal is chosen from competing alternatives.

An example of this process concerning a private problem coming to the attention of the policy-makers could be that of a man passionately concerned about the standards of midwifery or obstetric care after his wife has died in childbirth:

- With information about the standards of care, good networks and effective lobbying, he could raise his concern to another level so that it becomes a public concern
- Of the many public problems arising, only a few lead to the development of a health policy in order to attempt to solve the problem
- The next step is to get the problem onto the 'policy agenda'

- Then the problem must be turned into an issue. This happens when the public cannot agree on the best solution for the problem
- Therefore an issue has emerged that may or may not raise the interest of the policy-makers
- The policy-makers may choose or feel they have to act upon the issue because the bereaved man's private concern about the standards of midwifery care has become a public concern that the public cannot solve
- If the policy-makers choose the issue, the the need for improved standards of midwifery and obstetric care becomes part of the political agenda
- The approach described by Parsons above may then move into action
- Policies also need institutions and people who manage the implementation and the changes that are required. Getting involved in policy implementation is discussed below
- Policy formulation and implementation cannot always be separated because those developing the policy often have to adapt their proposals to what has to be done in order to gain acceptance
- Similarly, the policy analysis to identify the best alternative may be far too costly and is thus replaced by only a little analysis, other information and creativity.

Lindblom (1968) mentions some strategies used to develop policies for very difficult problems. Nurses can probably identify many of these strategies in the health policies that affect their work. These include:

1. *satisficing*, or not trying too hard, and agreeing to an acceptable solution rather than the best one
2. *a deliberate little mistake* made in a policy in order to avoid a big mistake: the little mistake can then be rectified with the next policy
3. *feedback* by creating policy enabling the policy analyst to get new answers and learn more in time about the problem and a better solution
4. *remediality*, resolving immediate problems and not thinking strategically
5. *seriality*, which is typically the never-ending process of policy-making in small incremental steps
6. *bottlenecking*, a process that happens automatically and by intent when the goal cannot easily be achieved; in order to have a reasonable excuse for failure, a bottleneck is created as a diversion.

Blunden and Dando (1994, p. 100) discussing Vickers' life work noted that Vickers described the ongoing process of health policy change as a kind of impossible necessity and at best a temporary resolution of priority issues – never a once and for all achievement and never a reachable goal. Instead, he claims that it is a goal-setting process with an attempt to find an acceptable place between new realities and the standards of acceptability, each of which alters with changing societal conditions, events and perceptions. The understanding of what is and what ought to be in an issue (that the public cannot solve) triggers the regulatory policy mechanisms.

A number of health care policies collected together could be the framework for a health system. This health system is not necessarily a structure but a collection of policies, processes and activities by which people in a locality or health sector, acute, community or general practice setting receive their care. The collections of policies that make up a health system are part of the real world, which is complex, chaotic and a much larger environment. That environment affects both health systems and their associated policies. Those studying, analysing or wishing to influence policies have to find time to analyse and interpret what is going on in the environment. Unfortunately, this environment is fluid, dynamic and often difficult to grasp. In addition, any one policy decision is made within a web of decisions and politics, and a decision in one area will most probably affect policies in other areas. There is also of course a two-way flow between the health system and the environment. Describing this complex reality does not make policies any easier to study or interpret, but the nurse who is trying to understand, interpret, implement or develop a health policy has nevertheless to understand the policy process, the health system and the interaction with the environment.

Frenk (1994) describes four levels of policy processes in the health system:

1. The *systematic level* is the one that shapes the health system overall; Acts of Parliament or Policies of Congress fall into this category
2. The *programmatic level* decides the priorities for health care, the nature of the provision and how the resources will be allocated. One example is the local development of policies to support specific groups such as elderly frail patients
3. The *organisational level* is where policies are developed about the way in which the business will operate, both financially and qualitatively. Policies at this level could be those governing the contractual relationships between providers and purchasers

4. *Instrumental level* policies are concerned with how the organisation is managed in order to achieve organisational goals. Instrumental policies may ensure that policies at other levels are implemented.

Health systems and government

Health systems are closely allied to the government of any particular country. The composition of the health system of three of the countries covered in this book – the UK, the USA and Australia – will be considered.

The UK has one National Health Service (NHS) funded from taxation and led by a government department (DoH). In addition, there is a small and growing independent sector. The DoH is headed up by a Secretary of State, three Ministers of State (two in the House of Commons and one in the House of Lords) and a Parliamentary Under Secretary. Each of the Ministers and the Under Secretary has separate responsibilities, and in 1999 one of the Ministers of State had nursing included in the portfolio. The DoH has three responsibilities: public health, social care and the NHS Executive.

The NHS Executive's aims are to promote health, prevent ill-health, diagnose and treat injury and disease, and care for people who have a long-term disability with equity, efficiency and responsiveness. The role of the NHS Executive is to provide clear strategic leadership to NHS Trusts (providers) and health authorities (purchasers), as well as supporting the Ministers of Health in the development of public policies, securing resources through the Public Expenditure Survey and establishing a resource framework. The NHS Executive also attempts to improve the knowledge base of the service by accurately reflecting the most advanced understanding of what is clinically effective coupled with a systematic assessment of the actual health benefits received. Finally, it manages the NHS to ensure that policy is implemented. Within the above, key objectives are identified for the NHS Executive that are expected to make a year-on-year contribution to long-term health strategy (DoH, 1998).

The USA has a federal system of parliament in which the states have formed a unity but remain independent in internal affairs. The US federal government has certain specified powers, all other powers being retained by the 51 states. The Federal Department of Health and Human Services (HHS) is the US government's principal agency for protecting the health of all Americans and providing essential human services, especially for those who are unable to care for themselves. The HHS manages more than 300 programmes covering a wide spectrum of activities, for example medical and social science research, preventing outbreaks of disease, Medicare (health insurance for elderly and disabled Americans) and Medicaid (health insurance for people with a low income). The HHS works closely with the state and local governments. State or county agencies provide many of the HHS services at a local level. The US President appoints most positions in the HHS.

Each state of the USA has its own Department of Health. For example, the mission of the Department of Health in Washington State is to empower individuals and communities to make informed choices, to assure access to quality prevention and illness care, to protect people from environmental threats to their health and to advocate sound, cost-effective health policies. The state Governor appoints the Secretary of Health (Washington State Department of Health, 1998).

Australia also has a federal government. Australia's Commonwealth Department of Health and Family Services carries out a strategic role on behalf of the government, providing national leadership, setting national standards and targets, and purchasing health and family services. The Department is decreasing its role in direct service delivery and service management through a purchaser/provider split and, in the longer term, transferring some of the service purchasing functions to the state governments (Commonwealth Department of Health and Family Services, 1998). Both the USA and Australia have considerably more health insurance funding than the UK and in the USA a large amount of health care is managed by Health Maintenance Organizations (HMOs).

The way in which decisions are taken and developed into health policy and the manner in which the policies are developed differ markedly in each of these three countries. To a great extent, this is determined by the style of government. Decisions are taken in the USA federal government, for example in one of many committees, whereas in the UK, government decisions are taken in the one Cabinet. In the USA, although there are a large number of federal programmes for health, most policy decisions are made by the individual state Departments of Health and their regions. In the UK, the government's DoH sets the health policy direction for the four countries of England, Wales, Scotland and Northern Ireland. These four countries are now, however, taking increasing responsibility for the development of their own country's health policies. In England, the DoH has regional offices that oversee the health commissioning of the district health authorities and primary care groups in their geographical area. All countries are in a process of change, this currently being reflected in the catch-up contemporary health reform.

WHY SHOULD NURSES GET INVOLVED IN THE POLICY PROCESS?

The first part of the chapter provided an introduction to the rest of the book. The complexity of the policy process and the link between government and politics, policy development and the health system have been introduced. This next section takes the reader carefully through reasons why nurses should be involved in the policy processes and how to initiate or improve their skills in doing so.

The values of nursing

This enquiry cannot begin without reconsidering the fundamental values of nursing. 'Value' is a small yet multifaceted word, deriving its interpretation from its contextual use. It could have an association with utility, merit, bargain and worth or it could convey a meaning of amount or attribute (Dickenson-Hazard, 1997). Nurses may not always directly understand the durability of the values of nursing. In many instances, they have given them little thought since qualifying and are therefore not in a position to discuss them with any confidence at the negotiating table. Nevertheless, this is what is expected of nurses' contribution to the development of policy.

The values of nursing in the Western world are deeply rooted in Judaeo-Christian ethical values, as can be confirmed by reading the history of Florence Nightingale (Woodham-Smith, 1950), the founder of modern-day nursing. These values of nursing include a belief in:

> an equitable, universal health care service... which values the individual and the community; a service that acknowledges the... right to health care to meet – within realistic resource level – the... need for care, a service that respects their right to humane respectful... care and attention, and to protection from abuse and exploitation. (Swain, 1995, p. 8)

Nurses thus value health and those people who seek health. This leads nurses to learn how to keep people healthy and how to care.

There are both quantitative and qualitative values. The former have a monetary or numerical worth, the latter deeply intrinsic qualities that challenge measurement. Dickenson-Hazard (1997) suggests that, in the contribution that nurses make to health care, values should be humane, people-focused, knowledge-based, innovative and creative, politically astute and technologically and economically sound. Nurses also demonstrate compassion and reality. All these values comprise a mixture of humanitarianism and cost-effectiveness. In their everyday work caring for patients, nurses merge these values using sophisticated knowledge-gathering techniques and the unique models of decision-making, planning and evaluation of Parker and Wiltshire, described earlier in this chapter. Contemporary health care environments demand both humanitarian behaviour and rational cost-effective considerations. It is therefore important that both types of value are expressed in the policy processes. In order to influence health policy, nurses must use their experiences and demonstrate that they understand the economic factors and the degree of excellence required in health care.

In the evolution of our future society, the values that nursing supports are essential. At the start of the 21st century, the public are urging that society develop a new way of life, including more compassion and care for the most vulnerable people in the community. The public wants a humane society, the positive use of knowledge and technology and the maintenance of age-old religious expressions and institutions, as well as changes in all structures in society. Consideration for others, compassion and humanity will somehow have to be combined with the contemporary values of economics, individualism and knowledge. Nurses, the profession of nursing and its espoused values have much to offer the policy development that will determine the future health systems and society.

Although many nurses may consider that these values are currently politically and socially unacceptable, they are nevertheless the very values that have formed their characters and led them to quite often very senior appointments. They are the enduring values of society formed through centuries and decades of nursing care. This history, therefore, cannot be dismissed, and they are indeed also the humanitarian values for which society is searching. A precursor for a humane nursing service and a humane society is the acknowledgement of the humanity of each and every one of us. The last point of course encompasses not only the unique characters of all those whom nurses serve, but also the unique part that each individual nurse plays in the health system.

Environmental, organisational and clinical issues in contemporary situations

The essential contribution that nurses can and must make to policy development on executive and decision-making committees such as health boards has been the subject of much research and many papers and documents (Robinson and Strong, 1987; DoH, 1992; WHO, 1992; Hennessy *et al.*, 1993; Hennessy and Gilligan, 1994). Indeed, Hennessy and Wall (1996) have urged nurses on executive boards to demonstrate their added value to the board by advising on a wide range of subjects. These include commissioning health facilities and processes, making a contribution to national policy developments on care and keeping the executive boards informed about developments taking place in nursing nationally, in Europe and worldwide.

Nurses are expected to reflect those issues which have emerged as a result of their clinical experiences, clinical links and the philosophical stance of nursing, but nurses do not always do so. Quite often, they do not participate as much as they ought to, simply because of perceived competition with the voice of the medical lobby or the reality of cost restrictions. This is sometimes due to the dulling of sensitivity over time, the overload of work and the increasing importance of peer relationships over and above the needs of patients. There may also be the difficulty of articulating the breadth and complexity of nursing in fast-moving and competitive environments. Perhaps, then, one should not be surprised at this situation, which is considered by Hennessy and Swain (1997a, pp. 3–4):

> In the past decade there has been a gradual eroding of the professional confidence of many of those who work in clinical practice within the NHS, certainly, and especially, among nurses. The values, too, which many espouse are felt to be disregarded and considered by others to be old-fashioned.

This situation has developed since the introduction of general management into the UK and many other countries, with progressive attempts to eliminate perceived restrictive professional practices thought to be outdated and ineffective, either financially or clinically. The original policy was surely introduced to benefit patients rather than to exclude the voices of the professional group who had first-hand experience of patient needs. There is a constant flow of publications discussing morale within clinical professional groups, the importance of their relationship with managers and the need for professionals to improve their approach to new policy objectives (Harrison and Pollitt, 1994; Hennessy, 1995).

Changes in the labour market, technology and financial resources are also diluting professionals' control and influence over health care decisions. An example of this is the financial contracts for health care that frequently limit the activities of professionals. A nurse working in the community may be required to care for a discharged patient for no longer than a certain number of days, in agreement with the contract between the commissioner and the provider. The professional opinion of the nurse, however, may be that the patient is not ready to be discharged.

There is also increasing skill substitution and professional boundary-blurring (Pew Health Professions Commission, 1995; Institute of Medicine, 1996; NHS Confederation, 1997). These policy developments in the health care environment challenge the way in which nurses see themselves, their self-esteem and the value that they set on their own knowledge and ability. These changes also offer numerous opportunities. For example, the rise of the advanced clinical nurse and the nurse practitioner in many countries has given some nurses more skill, status and confidence.

Professional obligation

Nurses can gain much personally, first from the privilege and satisfaction that comes from caring for people when they are sick and dependent, and second, from their educational preparation to become a nurse. This is especially so because they also belong to:

> an occupation that requires advanced education and involves intellectual skills. (*Collins Dictionary*, 1978)

Harris and Holm (1997, p. 625) state that:

> It is usually assumed that a professional status includes both privileges (exclusive rights to perform certain actions) and obligations. The obligations are often formalised in a professional code of ethics, which has usually been formulated by the profession.

The UKCC has formulated the *Code of Professional Conduct for the Nurse, Midwife and Health Visitor* for the UK. For some years, this code has provided a statement of the values of the nursing professions and establishes the framework within which nurses, midwives and health visitors practise and conduct themselves. It puts a clear responsibility on all professional nurses to:

ensure that no acts or omission on his or her part or within his/her sphere of influence is detrimental to the condition or safety of patients or clients. (UKCC, 1992a, para. 2)

The Code also says that, in the exercise of professional accountability, nurses shall:

Have regard for the environment of care and its physical, psychological and social effects on patients/clients... and make known to appropriate persons or authorities any circumstances that could place patients/clients in jeopardy. (UKCC,1992a, para. 10)

In 1992, the UKCC published *The Scope of Professional Practice*. This stated:

Once registered, each nurse, midwife, or health visitor remains subject to the Code and ultimately accountable to the Council (UKCC) for his or her acts and omissions. This position applies regardless of the employment circumstances and regardless of whether individuals are actively engaged in practice. (UKCC, 1992b, para. 5.5)

These three paragraphs make it quite clear that nurses are expected to use their knowledge and get involved in political processes for the safety and benefit of their patients.

Harris and Holm (1997) indicate that there are risks associated with professional obligations. The existence of a moral and public-interest argument for 'nurses to make known to persons or authorities any circumstances that could place patients/clients in jeopardy' may be risky to the nurse's employment or contractual status. This has been particularly so over the past decade during which competition between health providers has been encouraged, as an employee who exposes unmet health needs may cause embarrassment to his or her employing organisation. This situation creates tension between the moral obligation of a professional nurse and his or her accountability to the employer. This may be one reason why nurses do not appear to be using their knowledge and experience of patients' needs and engaging in health policy work as much as they should in order to meet their professional obligations.

As recently as 1997 in the UK, Fursland reported that any nurse who 'blew the whistle' on bad practice still risked the tenure of his or her job and promotion prospects. The Public Interest Disclosure Bill (House of Commons, 1997) should lead to legislation that would protect health service employees if they expose malpractice.

An accumulated body of knowledge

Nurses have a large body of knowledge accumulated through their basic and continuing education. More importantly, however, there is the understanding of patients and their needs that arises from nurses' direct experience of caring for patients (Parker and Wiltshire, 1997). Nursing care is given to people of all ages, creeds, ethnic groups and social status. The care is often personal and of a very intimate nature. While nurses practise the art and science of nursing, their patients, and sometimes the patients' carers and families, talk about their hopes, fears and pain. In turn, nurses listen to what is said so that they can learn what care their patients need. In addition, they find out how patients are responding and what they think about the care that is being provided. This very important two-way communication attempts to ensure that the nursing care given is appropriate and relevant for each patient. There are, of course, limiting factors such as the nature of the illness and limited resources.

Of all health care professionals, nurses have a very special and frequently much longer relationship with patients. This is because nurses or midwives are usually present at a patient's *first* contact with the health system, for example, on admission to the accident and emergency department following a trauma or to the labour ward for a new birth. Nurses support and care for those patients and their families who require short spans of treatment, as well as others who need very long periods of care. Many of the latter are the more vulnerable people in society, such as the very aged, the mentally ill or disabled, and those with chronic and degenerative disabilities. Nurses are frequently present during the patient's discharge from the health system at the end of an episode of care, and are sometimes there at the bedside at the end of life. In this situation, many other health care professionals may walk away and leave the nurse to care for the bereaved relatives as well as the patient's body.

The close relationships that nurses have with their patients also expose the more fundamental problems underlying ill-health, their roots lying in factors such as anxiety, broken relationships, poverty, deprivation, unemployment and bad or no housing. Nurses working in the community meet these in face-to-face situations. Nurses also understand the environment of health care – health and financial targets, efficiency, purchasers, planning, delivery, health provision contracts, service specifications and quality.

Over time, nurses' many and varied experiences become a sound body of knowledge about patients and their families' health and care needs, and about how these should be met within resources available. It could thus be expected that nurses would believe they have a moral responsibility to use this knowledge for the common good. Similarly, it could also be anticipated that nurses would be fully involved and have considerable influence over social and health policies that improve the life and welfare of the public.

This intimate knowledge is accepted much more readily in the policy arena if nurses use the opportunity to back up their experiences either with their own collated and analysed clinical data or by making use of epidemiological data and research evidence (Mulhall, 1996).

DO NURSES HAVE MORE INFLUENCE THAN THEY RECOGNISE?

Christine Hancock, General Secretary of the UK's Royal College of Nursing (RCN), believes that nurses possess much more influence than they give themselves credit for (Hancock, 1997). This is despite the fact that nurses often face difficult struggles when trying to demonstrate to others the value of nursing. This is compounded because so much of nurses' work is undetected and takes place away from the public eye. There is also the age-old problem of sexual discrimination against a predominately female profession. Hancock states that nurses understand the reality of patient care and this is why people listen to them. If this is really true, why do we hear again and again that nurses feel thwarted, undervalued and powerless?

A number of chapters in this book describe the positive influence that nurses have had on influencing policy (see Chapters 2, 3 and 7). Others show gaps in the achievements of nursing despite great efforts by the profession, as described by Walsh and Gough (Chapter 13). Birt, in Chapter 5, points out that his experience in the European public health arena demonstrates that nurses are not using all the opportunities offered to them.

Over the past few years, I have worked with many nurses, in very senior positions and from a number of countries, who are striving to influence health and social policies for the benefit of their patients' health. Generally speaking, these same nurses believe that they are not as successful in their endeavours as they would like to be. In many cases, it is obvious that these senior nurses recognise that they have knowledge and skills to offer the policy processes, and want to use them, but *fail to recognise* the signs of the times. By this, I mean that nurses frequently do not see the bigger picture, the policy opportunities and the interconnections between different policies. They also

simply have little experience in networking, lobbying and how to focus
on the critical issues.

This may be because, in the recent past, many governments have had
a more patriarchal style of management and less delegated decision-
making and consultation. The population, and nurses as part of that
population, may therefore have had less of a role in the development
and implementation of policy. Nowadays, however, most countries have
changed their way of working to not only a more democratic style, but
also a position in which much of the decision-making takes place
nearer to those affected by the policies. This is happening in the UK, the
government setting the principles of the direction and local purchasers
being responsible for providing health care in a locally determined way.
This approach is similar to that of the federal governments described in
both the USA and Australia. Hence, nurses who work so closely with
patients will simply have to get involved in the development and implementation of social and health policies. Actually to get involved
requires an understanding of how to do so. The text that follows should
begin to broaden our comprehension of the subject. The subsequent
chapters will also provide many examples.

HOW TO GET INVOLVED

Focusing on the right issues in nursing policy

The work of nurses is clearly linked to politics and the political system
through the health system and health policies within which nursing
is practised. It is difficult to know the limits of the territory of nursing
policy because nursing care covers such a wide range of activities,
patient care groups and care settings. In addition, nurses have such
relevant real experiences with patients and health care provision.
They possess a very immediate and recent knowledge as well as an
accumulated history of knowledge. It is hard to know which subjects
to choose at a particular time, which to tackle at a later date and
which to leave out, even if the latter are important. If one tries to
tackle too much, very little is achieved. A critical issue chosen is often
not a single entity but part of a bigger picture or whole network of
interrelated policies.

Nursing is also a richly diverse profession, nurses themselves being
derived from many different backgrounds and beliefs. This demonstrates a plurality of approach, which also happens in the nursing
care process and leads to an important fusion, or synthesis, of scien-

tific, ethical, moral and caring human values. Although all this re-emphasises the importance of nurses being fully involved with the policy processes, it simultaneously demonstrates one of the difficulties that nurses face when they try to identify the important issues. There is so much to do and nurses have so many real-life experiences that they frequently find it extraordinarily difficult not to be overwhelmed by the magnitude of the issues that they could tackle. For the same reason, it may also be particularly difficult to focus on the most important issues. These are especially those which will both be accepted by other politically influential people and also have the most benefit for health gain.

Agenda-setting

This is the process used to turn an ideological issue into a policy proposal. Parsons (1955, p. 115) used 'sleeping in the streets' as an example of an issue for agenda-setting. Sleeping on the streets could be understood as a problem related to homelessness, so policies could be developed to provide housing for the homeless. Of course, the problem of sleeping on the streets could be more complex and connected to other issues, addictive behaviour being only one example. An agenda could then be set to develop policies related to both the housing and rehabilitation of those with addictive behaviour who slept on the streets. Another example about midwifery and obstetric care is used earlier in the chapter when considering policy formulation.

An important documented example of agenda-setting in nursing is that of two papers by Kitson *et al.* (1997a, b). These papers outline the development of an agenda to influence policy in health care research. One describes using an explicit agenda-setting or policy-making model described by Lomas (1993a), which was used to establish a co-ordinated and systematic method for identifying priorities for research and development in nursing. This model was also used to consider how nursing was influencing the contemporary national clinical effectiveness and research policy work. Consideration was given to whether a priority-setting exercise could make a difference to the wider health services research agenda.

Finally, the agenda-setting model of Sabatier and Mazmanian (1980) is described by Murphy in Chapter 8 of this book. She describes how this model was used to influence the national nursing education policy in Canada.

Mapping the environment and process of policy development and implementation

Experience has demonstrated that it is helpful to try to map the policy environment. When the system and environment have been mapped or modelled, individuals can use them to clarify the processes and the interactions that could, or should, happen in policy development and implementation. It will also assist in identifying the potential sources of both positive and negative influences.

The mapping process can be used retrospectively to understand the results of the development and implementation of a health policy process. This can provide insight into outputs, outcomes and the effects of the event, providing interesting and sometimes essential feedback. The model below has been developed with the help of many experienced nurses attending health policy seminars (Hennessy, 1998). It was adapted from a model developed by Lomas (1993b) to describe the implementation of policies based on research evidence relating to the clinical area. The Hennessy model exposes the truth that any policy or health system is within, and affected by, all that is happening in the wider environment.

There are a number of domains, or spheres of influence to consider in the mapping process. These are not mutually exclusive, actually merging haphazardly into each other. To make the process easier to understand and use, a number of domains have been identified (Figure 1.1).

1. *Knowledge and information.* This includes the development of the policy subject through identification of need, lobbying, consultation, research and new information.
2. *Social.* The social domain covers the impact of society on any policy. If the policy to be implemented is less important than other issues in the social domain, it may be difficult to get acceptance and support from the local community. A good example of this is the lack of support that may occur when a hospital attempts, even for very sound reasons, to reduce the number of inpatient beds: the local community may not accept these reasons.
3. *Consumer.* The attitudes, knowledge and expectations of the public have an increasingly important impact on both the development and the implementation of policy. Government policy in some countries strongly encourages the public to get involved. Sometimes they do, and then frequently sway the policy processes. On other occasions, it is hard to get the public involved and even harder to get an objective opinion.

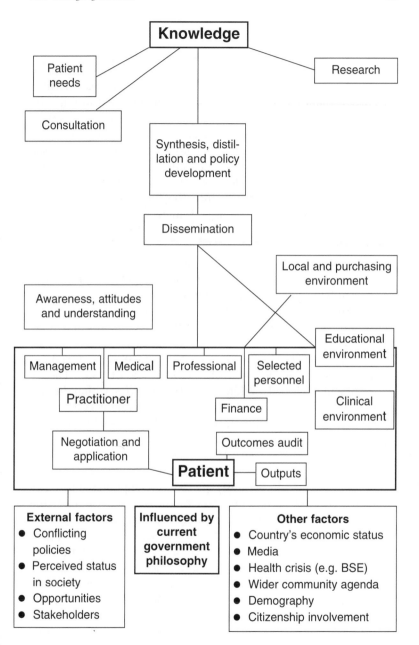

Figure 1.1 Policy implementation in the clinical environment

4. *Education.* The role of education is extremely important in dissemination and assists with changing attitudes and the management of change that may be necessary to implement a policy.
5. *Clinical environment.* The environment within which care takes place is strongly influenced by the style of management, the way in which change is managed, the contractual and financial constraints, the roles and interaction of the professionals and the actual relationships between patients and clinicians. It becomes clear from Figure 1.1 that if the communication systems are inadequate within the clinical environment, the implementation of policies can be seriously compromised. It is well known that policy documents do not automatically find their way into the hands of clinicians. In nursing, national figures and organisations such as the UK's Chief Nursing Officer, the RCN and the UKCC all go to great lengths to ensure that important policies affecting nursing are well disseminated. This is achieved with varying success and can be quickly monitored by tracing the dissemination route of a specific policy and identifying any blockages that have occurred.
6. *Purchasing environment and local environment.* Health and social care purchasers disseminate and influence policies and their implementation.
7. *Current government philosophy.* The philosophy of the government has a massive influence on health policies. The UK's new Labour government published a White Paper, *The New NHS,* within the first 6 months of election. Despite the major health reforms introduced by the previous government, the White Paper stated that it was poised to 'modernise the National Health Service to meet the demands of the public' (DoH, 1997, p. 3).
8. *National issues.* The development and implementation of health policies are frequently seriously affected or compromised by other national priorities, two examples being the economic status of the country and the changing demography of the population.
9. *Other external factors.* Other factors could include conflicting policies, the perceived status of the policy, the views of important stakeholders and windows of opportunity. At times, a policy emerges that appears to conflict with an earlier one. Those with the responsibility for its implementation then try to resolve the conflict or manage the two policies in a creative way. They may ask for clarification from those who created the policy, yet the latter have usually not realised that there are conflicting issues.

In addition, there are subjects that do not attract the attention of others. Unfortunately, there are policies that, although very important for the good health of the nation, may not appeal to the larger public – usually those which are associated with more vulnerable populations and less powerful professionals. An example of this is policies linked to the nursing care of people who are elderly, frail and mentally ill.

Walt (1994) described macro politics as that which matters to everyone and micro politics as that which involves more localised and sectoral interests. Many issues that concern nurses are localised, but nurses can and do on occasions bring these into the wider arena and attract the attention of those involved in the macro policy process (Hennessy, 1997). A good example of the latter is perhaps the dogged attempts of nurses to raise the profile and importance to the public of the use of nurse practitioners to carry out the more routine and time-consuming medical tasks. These tasks include technical procedures, prescribing and health and patient education.

Stakeholders have a very important role in the creation and implementation of a policy. Politicians, well-known local figures or influential clinicians are well placed to persuade a majority either to support or to block a policy process. Many nurses garner considerable support for issues that concern them. For some subjects, a chief nurse may be more likely to be listened to by policy-makers than may a professional nurse in a position closer to the patient, although on occasions the reverse may be true.

Policies that are implemented sometimes do not appear to be very important. They may, however, have had the benefit of very powerful supporters, or the policy-maker may have had another agenda that is not immediately obvious. Consider, for example, the introduction of the 'named nurse' approach in 1991. For many outside the nursing profession, this may not have been a very important development. For patients, it could have been particularly comforting to know who their nurse was, and a proportion of nurses were very satisfied. The concept, however, was very difficult to implement in certain clinical areas such as acute care, where nurses work shifts and the patients' length of stay is continuously decreasing. This means that the patient's 'named nurse' may not even be on duty for most of the patient's inpatient stay. All of these factors could be considered in advance when policies are created – but often are not.

Mapping the policy process as described in these paragraphs clarifies what is happening, what should happen and the part that the individual nurse could have in the process.

INFLUENCING THE DEVELOPMENT OF POLICIES

As has already been mentioned several times, the wisdom of nurses, developed through their clinical experiences, and their intimate knowledge of those for whom they care should be articulated at all levels of the policy processes. This information is best expressed in the policy arena when supported by the nurses' own clinical data or existing research evidence or epidemiological data.

There are some very interesting examples of the influence that the nursing profession has had on policy nationally. For example, in 1986 the profession insisted that community nursing be reviewed when primary care was being reviewed, prior to the publication of the Green Paper on primary care (DHSS, 1986a). This led to *Neighbourhood Nursing* (DHSS, 1986b) and the inclusion of a summary of this report in the Green Paper (DHSS, 1986a). A similar situation developed in 1997 when the RCN insisted that nursing have a higher profile in the White Paper *The New NHS* (DoH, 1997). This may have encouraged the government's previous expression of interest to increase the role of nurses in primary care. To fulfil this objective, they included nurses in the proposals for primary care groups, which replaced general practice fundholders as the lead body in the new NHS in April 1999. Many other examples can be found over the past decade of where nurses have attempted to influence national policy development by focusing on the role that the nursing profession has in a specific subject area. An example of this is *The Nursing, Midwifery and Health Visiting Contribution to the Health of the Nation* (DoH, 1993a).

There are other good examples of every effort being made by the professions to be proactive and influence pending legislation, for example urging health authorities to seek advice from suitable persons in the professions, including nursing, about appropriate commissioning for the care of patients. This was included in an executive letter and shortly afterwards incorporated into the 1995 Health Authorities Act (DoH, 1995a).

It is of great interest that, despite the efforts of the profession to get this particular point enshrined in legislation, it could still not be enough. A nurse in a primary care group, however, will be in a position to influence commissioning. There seems to be a general consensus that the nursing contribution to corporate strategy development is weak (Hennessy, 1998), that much professional advice given is on an *ad hoc* basis and that nurses are seldom formally asked for professional advice (NHS Executive, Northern and Yorkshire,

1996). This is another lesson. Once an issue has become a policy influence, it is still very important to ensure that the policy is implemented and then evaluated in order to measure its impact.

Getting the message heard

The attention that issues receive will depend on the importance of the impact of the subject and the vociferousness of those trying to attract attention. Making more noise does not necessarily mean that one is more likely to be listened to or heard. Issues sometimes receive attention because they raise questions about power and legitimacy. At other times, issues that one party thinks are important may be squeezed out of the policy process as they are perceived by others not to be priorities or because the people who are lobbying, or for whom they are lobbying, do not have sufficient power (Barker, 1996). Important issues sometimes do not reach the policy arena simply because the people who are developing the policies do not perceive the issues to be important or do not realise that they are important. As in the case of neglecting to introduce policies that ensure the safety of patients or staff, this can and does have disastrous consequences. Another example of this is the dilatory introduction of policies concerning new infectious diseases alongside an outbreak of an epidemic that could have been prevented with the correct policies in place.

In order to get a message heard, a very important starting point is to feel passionately about the subject. An emotional, inarticulate message is not advocated. Instead, influence requires that the chosen subject is carefully considered and that the supporters are fired with enthusiasm. This should enhance the good data and evidence, planning, agenda-setting and networking with those others who have a knowledge of the subject. Networking is such an important aspect that it is discussed more fully later in this chapter. The policy strategy process has to be managed, with constant review and a change of direction when necessary, as managing a process does not automatically mean that it will be logical and straightforward. The process normally requires alertness, patience, determinism and constant review. Attention should be given to the important stakeholders. Pressure groups of persons with similar interest can be very useful in getting the message across. The medical profession are very successful in this regard and are usually heard. They can be foes or allies to the nursing voice, depending on the circumstances and whether doctors perceive that the nurses' power and position will be in any way challenging to the medical profession.

Using opportunities

Alertness and lateral thinking will assist in identifying many opportunities for policy involvement as they arise. In nursing, a few obstacles may have to be overcome, including competition *within* the profession that may compromise the development of a cohesive voice that would make a very powerful lobbying tool. There is also a cultural lag within the profession, descending from times when the profession was very hierarchical. In the past, the profession did not encourage its members to use the available opportunities for getting involved with policy processes; instead, nurses have been burdened with heavy caseloads of direct patient care, leaving the policy processes to others.

Although there are numerous opportunities for nurses to become involved in the policy processes, these are not always obvious and are very different from those of a few years ago. James, in a challenging description of the different styles of management in the NHS, suggests that earlier styles arose for the benefit of the professionals and the bureaucrats rather than the patients (James, 1994). Nevertheless, in the previous structures, nurses had a statutory position at all levels of bureaucratic management so clear responsibilities and the opportunities for influencing policies could have been more explicit. It would also have been easier to control, through top-down styles, the implementation of policy through the line management structure. Top-down styles have been described (Parsons, 1955) as being rigid, implementation occurring because of deference to the regulations. Recently, Robinson, during an interview (Parker, 1997), described a continuum of power in nursing with influence at one end, domination at the other and authority in between. Nurses, Robinson suggested, are not very good at influencing but are instead good at dominating or being dominated. This description fits the top-down management styles of a past era. Nowadays, the management style is generally more consultative, the expectation being that there will be a more bottom-up influential approach, with flexibility and a consideration of patient needs.

Although the previous management structures accommodated the general way in which nurses approached policy processes as described by Robinson, nurses do not seem to have been noticed as being particularly influential and are not often mentioned in general public policy textbooks (Thurber, 1991; Smith, 1993; Hill, 1997).

When analysing the successful introduction of a policy, one can frequently trace the use of a 'window of opportunity'. For example, the successful introduction of a no-smoking policy might be launched simultaneously with the publication of new research evidence demonstrating the incidence of lung cancer among smokers. It is not uncommon for nurses to react negatively when a new policy is introduced without looking for or noticing a 'window of opportunity' that may emerge. The varied approach to the 'New Deal' (NHSME, 1994), or the introduction of shorter working hours for junior doctors, led to much excitement as well as grumbling. On the one hand, nurses reacted, perhaps justifiably, to taking on more work without the financial rewards; on the other hand, a number of nurses excitedly took on new skills and roles.

Networks

An important key in the use of influence, which has probably only recently been given much attention by nurses, is the use of networks and pressure groups.

Networks of people with similar interests can become interest and pressure groups, which raise a mutually shared passion for specific issues. On occasions, interest groups form for an express purpose, such as the prevention of the closure of a much-loved hospital, that of St Bartholomew's Hospital in London during the 1990s being a case in point. Some interest groups may develop passions that are to the disadvantage of the public and of concern only to the members. Wilson (1990) believes that this usually happens when the group members are inadequately informed, whereas if they had adequate knowledge, the outcome could be for the common good. This is a lesson for policymakers to be open and honest in their consultation, and for nurses to do their best to gather adequate and accurate information to support their case. It cannot generally be said that all networks and interest groups have the aim of working for the common good as in many situations they are working for local, sectoral or even professional interest rather than for the benefit of the public. Networks and interest groups differ markedly in their structure, the way in which they function, their duration and their impact. The influence of networks does not only depend on the subject and the combined power of the members: the broad context within which they operate also has a marked influence. For example, a pressure group can only influence the government if the government chooses to listen. The influence is not only from the resources but from the historical, ideological and structural context within which they operate (Smith, 1993).

Policy networks can become powerful over time, especially by creating mutual and regular dialogue with influential stakeholders. They are particularly powerful if they possess information that the stakeholders need for the policy formation or implementation. Thurber (1991) claims that, in the UK, the state is highly dependent on professional knowledge for both the development and the implementation of health policy. Disappointingly, he also claims that this mutually acceptable relationship has traditionally existed between the state and the medical profession. Together they have created health policy, finding little need for other parties and almost totally excluding other health professionals. In the past decade, government policy has been changing this position and has developed a strong relationship between management networks and government, reducing the relationship with doctors. With this in mind, nurses may now be even further from the negotiating and influencing tables.

Professional interest groups can also be insider or outsider groups (Grant, 1989): the insider groups can access important stakeholders within minutes, whereas outsider groups may run campaigns and protests but still be denied access to the stakeholders. Networks can be local, national, pan-European or international. Examples of all the various types are mentioned in the chapters that follow.

EVALUATING – ANALYSING OR STUDYING THE POLICY
PROCESS RETROSPECTIVELY

This is usually left to the academics, few nurses taking the time to get involved. Mapping the process as described above is one very informative way of evaluating the implementation of policy and provides a wealth of rich material. It is also a very useful mechanism for learning how a policy was developed and what its effect has been. Hill (1997) makes four points about studying the process:

1. It will be appreciated that a policy process is normally a sequence of events, not necessarily logical, with little scope for comparisons with earlier models.
2. Any analysis is likely to be an individual case study, using qualitative methods. Impact analysis could, however, be quantitative and lead to comparative studies.
3. Analysts have to use methods involving inference from accessible data, one reason being that so much of the political process is secret. This is, however, not the only reason; in addition, in this kind of

evaluation, so much of the information received depends on the co-operation of those from whom the analyst is trying to extract the data and their willingness to provide accurate facts and figures.
4. Alternative courses of action that could have taken place could be explored, or the organisational process and behaviour as well as the reactions to the policy analysed.

A policy evaluation example in nursing is the process undertaken by two Chief Nursing Officers of the Department of Health. In 1988, the Chief Nursing Officer, Mrs (now Dame) Anne Poole produced a *Strategy for Nursing*. Mrs (now Dame) Yvonne Moores, her successor, launched a sequel called *A Vision for the Future* in 1993 (DoH, 1993b). The impact of this overall strategy has been continually evaluated, the first report being published in 1995 in a document called *Testing the Vision* (DoH, 1995). In 1998, a health services circular (HSC 1998/045, issue date 28 April) consulted on the next strategy for nursing and a new Nursing, Midwifery and Health Visiting Strategy will be published during 1999.

CONCLUSION

The movement of health care into and out of a market system in the UK and health reform in most other countries requires nurses to become more involved in the politics, economics and policy development of health care. In this respect, it should be noted that the White Paper, *The New NHS* (1997) has led to a dismantling of the NHS internal market and a move towards co-operation and contestability.

The following chapters raise many questions about how far nurses have travelled in this area. Ride in Chapter 4 develops a philosophical discussion about the possibility of an international nursing policy. Fawcett-Henesy (Chapter 6) describes how nurses have influenced policies about clinical developments in many countries in Europe. Similarly, Kearney and Redmond in Chapter 7 describe influence in one clinical area in many countries in the European Union (EU). Keighley in Chapter 9 discusses the impact of policy on nursing education in Europe, whereas Fry describes the implementation at a more local level of community care policies. The remaining chapters have been mentioned earlier. In summary, the book covers the views of a range of people including international policy-makers, public health doctors, nurses working in different world regions and continents, nurse educationalists, nurse researchers, health service researchers and nurses in executive positions.

In this chapter, the discussions cover the meaning of health policy, including the history and depth of policy processes. It is suggested that nurses should get involved because of their knowledge and its importance for patients, health care and their professional obligations. Methods of improving techniques for involvement and influence are covered in some depth. The content is therefore highly relevant to all nurses in policy positions and all nurses in postgraduate courses, especially in Europe. The following chapters will also be extremely useful to educationalists and their students for all nursing courses that have an element of health and social policy in the curriculum.

REFERENCES

Andersen, J. (1984) *Public Policy-Making*, 3rd edn. New York: CNS College Publishing.

Barker, C. (1996) *The Health Care Policy Process*. London: Sage.

Benzeval, M., Judge, K. and Whitehead, M. (1995) *Tackling Irregularities in Health: An Agenda for Action*. London: King's Fund.

Blunden, M. and Dando, M. (eds) (1994) *Rethinking Public Policy*. Wiltshire: Cromwell Press.

Campbell, A. (1984) *Moderated Love. A Theology of Professional Care*. London: SPCK.

Commonwealth Department of Health and Family Services (1998) http://www.health.gov.au/hfs-abt.htm.

Davies, L. (1995) *Gender and the Professional Predicament in Nursing*. Buckingham: Open University Press.

Department of Health (1988) *A Strategy for Nursing*. London: HMSO.

Department of Health (1992) *One Year On: The Nurse Director Post*. London: HMSO.

Department of Health (1993a) *The Nursing, Midwifery and Health Visiting Contribution to the Health of the Nation*. London: HMSO.

Department of Health (1993b) *A Vision for the Future*. London: HMSO

Department of Health (1995a) *The Health Authorities Act*. London: HMSO.

Department of Health (1995b) *Testing the Vision*. London: HMSO.

Department of Health (1997) *The New NHS*. London: Stationery Office.

Department of Health (1998) About the Department, available from http://www.doh.gov.uk/dhhome.htm.

Department of Health and Social Security (1986a) *Primary Health Care: An Agenda for Action*. A Green Paper. London: HMSO.

Department of Health and Social Security (1986b) *Neighbourhood Nursing: A Focus for Care* (Chairman: J. Cumberlege). London: HMSO.

Dickenson-Hazard, N. (1997) Executive message. *Reflections* **23**(3): 6.

Donahue, M. (1996) *Nursing: the Finest Art*, 2nd edn. St Louis: Mosby Year Book.

Foucault, M. (1973) *The Birth of the Clinic: An Archaeology of Medical Precep-tion*, translated by A.M. Sheridan-Smith. London: Tavistock.

Frenk, J. (1994) Dimensions of health system reform. *Health Policy* **27**: 19–34.

Grant, W. (1989) *Pressure Groups, Politics and Democracy in Great Britain*. London: Philip Allan.

Hancock, C. (1997) People's contract, *Nursing Standard* **12**(5): 20.

Harris, J. and Holm, S. (1997) Risk-taking and professional responsibility. *Journal of the Royal Society of Medicine* **90**(11): 625–9.

Harrison, S. and Pollitt, C. (1994) *Controlling Health Professionals*. Buck-ingham: Open University Press.

Hennessy, D. (1995) Healthcare Professionals in the New NHS. *Focus* **1**: 3. Birm-ingham: Health Services Management Centre, University of Birmingham.

Hennessy, D. (1997) The shape of things to come. *Nursing Times* **23**(27): 36–8.

Hennessy, D.A. (1998) Information collected from participants of Health and Nursing Policy Seminars 1997/8 run by Developing Health Care. Canter-bury, Kent.

Hennessy, D.A. and Gilligan, J.H. (1994) Identifying and developing tomorrow's Trust nursing directors. *Journal of Nursing Management* **2**: 37–45.

Hennessy, D. and Wall, A. (1996) Personal information gathered in workshops for nurse executives at the University of Birmingham.

Hennessy, D. and Swain, G. (1997a) Developing community health care. In Hennessy, D. (ed.) *Community Health Care Development*. Basingstoke: Macmillan.

Hennessy, D. and Swain, G. (1997b) Epilogue. In Hennessy, D. (ed.) *Community Health Care Development*. Basingstoke: Macmillan.

Hennessy, D.A., Buckton, K. and Rowlands, H. (1993) The corporate role of the nursing director. *Journal of Nursing Management* **1**(4): 161–9.

Hill, M. (1997) *The Policy Process in the Modern State*, 3rd edn. London: Prentice Hall.

House of Commons (1997) Public Interest Disclosure Bill. House of Commons Bill Session. 1996–7:41. London: Stationery Office.

Institute of Medicine (1996) *Nursing Staff in Hospitals and Nursing Homes: Is it Adequate?* Washington DC: National Academy of Sciences.

James, A. (1994) *Managing to Care*. London: Longmans.

Kitson, A., McMahon, A., Rafferty, A.M. and Scott, E. (1997a) On developing an agenda to influence policy in health-care research for effective nursing: a description of a national R&D priority-setting exercise. *NT Research* **2**(5): 323–34.

Kitson, A., McMahon, A., Rafferty, A.M. and Scott, E. (1997b) High priority. *Nursing Times* **93**(42): 25–30.

Lindblom, C. (1968) *The Policy-making Process*.Englewood Cliff: NJ: Prentice Hall.

Lomas, J. (1993a) Making policy explicit. Legislative policy-making and lessons for developing practice guidelines. *International Journal of Technology Assessment in Health Care* **9**(1): 11–25.

Lomas, J. (1993b) Retailing research. *Milbank Quarterly* **73**(3): 439–71.

Moore, J. (1992) The incrementalists: preface. In Moore, J. (ed.) *Writers on Strategy and Strategic Management*. London: Penguin.

Mulhall, A. (1996) *Epidemiology, Nursing and Healthcare*. Basingstoke: Macmillan.

NHS Confederation (1997) *Towards the 21st Century. A Way Forward for the NHS. A Consultation Document*. Birmingham: NHS Confederation.

NHS Executive, Northern and Yorkshire (1996) Ensuring the Effective Involvement of Professionals in Health Authority Work. HSG(95)11. Unpublished project report.

NHS Management Executive (1994) *The New Deal: Plan for Action*. DoH. E.L. (94/17).

Parker, J. (1997) Conversation. Jane Robinson in conversation with Judith Parker. *Nursing Times* **4**(1): 66–8.

Parker, J. and Wiltshire, J. (1997) The handover: three modes of nursing practice knowledge. In Gray, R. and Pratt, R. (eds) *Scholarship in the Discipline of Nursing*. Melbourne: Churchill Livingstone.

Parsons, W. (1955) *Public Policy*. Aldershot: W. Elgar.

Percival, E. (1997) *Nurses Driving Policy*. John Durdin Oration Paper Series No. 2. Adelaide: Department of Clinical Nursing, University of Adelaide.

Pew Health Professions Commission (1995) *Critical Challenges: Revitalising the Health Care Professions for the Twenty First Century*. Third report of the Pew Health Professions Commission. San Francisco: USCF Center for the Health Professions.

Robinson, J. and Strong, P. (1987) *Professional Nursing Advice after Griffiths: An Interim Report*. Warwick: Nursing Policy Studies Unit.

Sabatier, P.A. and Mazmanian, D. (1980) The implementation of public policy: a framework for analysis. *Policy Studies Journal* **8**: 538–60.

Smith, M. (1993) *Pressure Groups and Policy-making*. Hertfordshire: Simon Schuster.

Swain, G.W. (1995) *Clinical Supervision: The Principles and the Process*. London: HVA.

Thurber, J.A. (1991) Dynamics of policy subsystems in American politics. In Cigher, A.J. and Loomis, A. (eds) *Interest Group Politics*, 3rd edn. Washington DC: Congressional Quarterly.

United Kingdom Central Council for Nursing, Midwifery and Health Visiting (1992a) *The Code of Professional Conduct for Nurses, Midwives and Health Visitors*. London: UKCC.

United Kingdom Central Council for Nursing, Midwifery and Health Visiting (1992b) *The Scope of Professional Practice*. London: UKCC.

Walt, G. (1994) *Health Policy: An Introduction to Process and Power*. London: Zed Books.

Washington State Department of Health (1998) available from http://www.hhs.gov/abau/profile.html.

Wilson, K. (1990) *Interest Groups*. Oxford: Basil Blackwell.

Winnicott, D. (1990) *The Maturation Process and the Facilitating Environment*. London: Kormac.

Woodham-Smith, C. (1950) *Florence Nightingale*. Edinburgh: Constable.

CHAPTER TWO

Influencing policy and the impact of health policy on nursing policy in the USA

Carole P. Jennings

Editors' Introduction

The chapter is introduced by a description of the US health care system and how this fits into the global changes seen in health care. This is followed by a discussion of the impact of current health policy on nursing practice and of a vision for a nursing policy response. A sound description of the health policy arena in the USA is provided. Powerful networks of nurses and effective grass-roots lobbying in the home states are shown to support the work of nurse leaders in Washington. Key nurses are encouraged to become legislators, and nurses raise funds to support their elections. The relationship between health policy and nursing policy in the USA provides a clear example of this interaction.

BACKGROUND

The US health care delivery system serves as the background for this chapter, which discusses how health policy shapes and even changes nursing policy in a country. Similarly, of course, nursing policy also contributes to the formulation of broader health policy initiatives. The relationship is mutually reinforcing and reciprocal.

The USA continues to spend an enormous amount on health care, approaching one trillion dollars in 1998 and accounting for 15 per cent of the gross national product, with per capita health spending estimated at $3701 in 1995, dramatically higher than Germany, the UK or Canada for the same period (see Table 2.1). Health care is big business and profit drives this industry just as it drives every other sector of American life.

Table 2.1   Per capita health spending in US dollars, 1985–95

	1985	1995
Germany	1175	2134
United Kingdom	685	1246
Canada	1244	2049
United States	1711	3701

Source: OECD, 1997

The US health care system is one founded on an employer-based, voluntary insurance model – there is no universal coverage and many payers (both public and private) exist along with a variety of providers. In such a context, businesses continue to bear the brunt of escalating health care costs. The voluntary insurance model has spawned different systems of payment and delivery including, most notably, managed care. Along with pressures from organised business to keep insurance premiums low, change in the USA is being driven by rising costs, the failure to provide coverage for all, consumer dissatisfaction and the increasing recognition that the country has poor life expectancy and high infant mortality despite high health care costs (see Table 2.2).

Table 2.2   Health outcome measures, 1995

	Infant Mortality*	Life expectancy at birth		Life expectancy at age 60	
		Men	Women	Men	Women
Germany	5.3	73.0	79.5	18.1	22.5
United Kingdom	6.2	74.3	79.7	18.3	22.4
Canada	6.3	75.3	81.3	19.9	24.3
United States	8.0	72.5	79.2	18.9	22.9

*Per 1000 live births
Source: OECD, 1997

Historically, health policy decisions, since the 1995 enactment of Medicare (health insurance for the disabled and those over the age of 65) and Medicaid (health insurance for the poor), have focused on cost containment strategies. Each strategy worked well for a limited period of time. Prospective payment and diagnostic related groups (DRGs) took the 'fat' out of hospital costs, the Resource Based Relative Value Scale (RBRVS) sought to appropriately adjust physician fees by setting up an elaborate fee schedule, although Marmour and Oberlander (1998) cite that 'the increase of market power to constrain physician practices and incomes – anticipated as possible outgrowths of Health Maintenance Organization (HMO) expansion – has proven in the 1990s to be far more dramatic than was expected'.

The growth of managed care, an approach that combines the financing and delivery of health care by providing for all necessary health care for an individual or group of individuals in exchange for fixed or 'capitation' payments has proceeded at a rapid pace. Today, some 160 million Americans – about 60 per cent of those with insurance – are in managed care plans, including an estimated 71 million in HMOs. Managed care is best seen as an array of techniques for containing costs and raising quality. Although managed care strategies are credited with reducing health care costs overall, policy analysts believe that cost savings attributed to managed care have levelled off, probaby in response to increased regulatory activity and current fierce market competition. Managed care 'tools', primarily the use of telemedicine to enhance access, greater use of guidelines and 'best practice' protocols, and expanded utilisation of non-physician providers (such as advanced practice nurses) are also proving to be of value to health care systems outside the USA.

Other palpable forces driving health policy decisions today include:

- the rise of corporate, investor-owned health care
- the movement of managed care into the public sector (Medicare and Medicaid programmes)
- the redefinition of the 'patient' as an informed consumer and customer
- the rapid diffusion of telecommunications technology (leading to significant forays into telehealth/telemedicine, long-distance learning applications, and sophisticated patient record systems that track an individual across an entire lifetime of service utilisation).

Technology is outpacing practice, and the technological imperative is placing a tremendous sense of urgency on the development of ethical guidelines and protocols. Additionally, cost is mediated by a more explicit concern with quality and value in health care services. Value judgements about health care are increasingly based on patient outcomes rather than cost or provider status.

INTRODUCTION

We begin the 21st century challenged, yet somewhat frightened and unsure of the next steps we should take. I would imagine that this 'fear' is normal and even useful. Hopefully, it has energised us and will continue to do so as we move ahead to adapt to, as well as shape the future of, health policy in our respective countries. As we work within our own borders and populations, we should realise that there are discernible forces reverberating internationally: the increasing resources required to accommodate the heavy demand for service; the ceaseless drive to relieve the burdens of illness, disability, and death; and the changing dynamic between individual accountability and social responsibility (Iglehart, 1991). Even though all nations face these same challenges, the dialogue needed to pursue the answers remains confined within our own geopolitical, cultural and economic environments.

Each health system represented today has its problems as well as its redeeming features. Those systems dominated by government decision-making and public finance long for more private resources and flexibility (examples of these systems being those of Canada and the UK), while those health care systems that allocate resources through private market-like mechanisms face pressures for more public-sector leadership and finance (the USA exemplifying this kind of system) (Iglehart, 1991). While the study of health care systems on a comparative basis is still in its infancy, we will move the process of comparative analysis forward as we simultaneously bring a mature and reasoned assessment of our own health care system and open our minds and philosophies (about how health care should be delivered and financed) to a broader understanding. I commend readers for their openness and vision. Health care needs are universal, and health care services continue to be a global commodity in great demand.

THE IMPACT OF CURRENT HEALTH POLICY TRENDS ON NURSING PRACTICE

Four interrelated characteristics of present day health care systems have significantly shaped and will continue to influence the practice of nursing in the USA. They provide the context for nursing education, research and practice today. These characteristics are: systemic change, interdependence, financial viability and the changing face of the health professions.

Systemic change

Health care systems worldwide cope with a common reality: they operate in a state of continuous change, striving to adjust to the economic, political and social demands of the moment. Health care reform in the USA is rapidly occurring at the federal, state and local levels. Each segment of government, along with the private sector, is faced with increasing costs, the need to expand access to necessary health services, and the ongoing assurance of quality in the services delivered.

Given the USA's penchant for reform, nurses have come to realise that the only predictable and stable parameter is change itself. They see the need proactively to embrace it and make a friend of it because change is all around. Our health care markets are increasingly driven by purchasers of health services, medical technology, medical supplies and pharmaceuticals. Certainly, in the USA, the market has spoken, and it says that the present system is too costly, is not performing well and has an enormous excess capacity in every respect – land, labour and capital. The often invisible hand of the market is driving the reform train, and American nurses do not want to continue to warm the seats at the station.

The main power-brokers in the US health care system today are the populations served, the providers of health care, including practitioners and institutions where care is delivered, suppliers such as pharmaceuticals and medical supply industries, private third-party payers, educational institutions that prepare health professionals, and the government as a regulator and sometimes payer (Hurst, 1991). All of these 'players' have undergone substantial change over the past 30 or so years. This constant of change is manifested by (Pew Health Professions Commission, 1995):

- the closure of half the hospitals in the USA and the resultant loss of 60 per cent of hospital beds
- a massive expansion of primary care in ambulatory and community settings
- a surplus of 100,000–150,000 physicians, as the demand for specialisation shrinks, a surplus of 200,000–300,000 nurses generated as hospitals close or restructure, and a surplus of 40,000 pharmacists as the dispensing function for drugs is automated and centralised
- the consolidation of many of the over 200 allied health professions into multiskilled professions as hospitals re-engineer their service delivery programmes

- an increased demand for public health professionals who can implement population-based interventions to meet the needs of a market-
  driven health care system
- a fundamental alteration of the health professional schools and the
  ways in which they organise, structure and frame their programmes
  of education, research and patient care.

In addition, integrated models for service delivery that literally
transport clients from womb to tomb have changed our basic perceptions about how and where care should be provided as well as how it
should be financed. This reality alone has produced tremendous
change within our present system as a whole and within the nursing
profession in particular.

Interdependence

Flowing from such change in our health sector is the move towards
increased interdependence – becoming interdependent partners in the
delivery of health services. The old 'team concept' has taken on fresh
perspective as health professions move away from parallel development, in which separate professional turfs were the accepted norm, to
an era of partnership and equality. The final arbiter for any service-
based system in the future must be the consumer of health care
services. In this context, professional turfs or prerogatives become
largely irrelevant as outcomes (and evidence-based practice), costs and
the health of populations drive the system.

The University of Maryland School of Nursing, as well as other
schools preparing professional nurses in the USA, is becoming increasingly multidisciplinary-sensitive. Nursing students are viewing their
care and contribution in the context of multidisciplinary team effort
and success. The use of critical pathways (which delineate the contribution of each team member to successful client outcomes) to guide
nursing practice is bringing us closer to the reality of interdependent
partners. As we write and implement new nursing curricula at the
University of Maryland, we hope to partner our nursing students with
medical, pharmacy, dental, physical therapy and social work students.
No longer can each profession operate in a vacuum.

Interdependence relates not only to a new collaboration between
health professionals, but also to a more appropriate relationship
between health care providers and the people they serve. Health
professionals must learn consumers' desires and expectations

regarding treatment outcomes – do they want more cure or care, high or low technology, access to alternative therapies? Providers must also depend on clients to report treatment outcomes and their satisfaction with the care they receive.

Financial viability

While American nurses disdain seeing health care productivity measured as the bottom line on a quarterly report, they are realising that the lifeblood of health care institutions and systems of care is financial viability. They know that financial viability must have meaning beyond short-term financial goals: it has to translate into long-term goals for the health of individuals, populations and the environments where people live, work, and spend their leisure time. Nurses are becoming well versed in economics, especially health economics, and are learning how to respond to hard economic questions and concerns with client-centred answers.

Nurses in the USA are working for healthy cities, increased health promotion and disease-prevention activities, supportive care for chronic and terminal illnesses and disability, patient/client education and enhanced consumer satisfaction and participation – all in the belief that cost, quality and value can coexist in the same context. In fact, lesser cost services can, in some situations, actually produce better outcomes and be of greater value to the client. 'Value' becomes a better construct when talking about quality and cost because it also includes care outcomes and consumer satisfaction. Nurses can and do indeed add 'value' to any medical intervention or health care experience.

The changing face of the health professions

The US health professions are changing as they realise that the system will not continue to support the health care labour force as it currently exists. The Pew Health Professions Commission (1995) directs nursing in the USA to implement the 'clinical management role' especially in relation to the advanced practice nurse with a Master's or doctoral degree. As clinical managers, nurses will help clients to negotiate the transitions between hospital, home and community, as well as across providers, to ensure the continuity as well as the cultural appropriateness of care.

The institutions in which health professionals are educated and the settings in which they work after graduation are urged to shift away from a supply-side orientation towards a demand-driven system (Pew Health Professions Commission, 1995). Supply will not continue to drive demand. In fact, the opposite will occur and will create challenges to the way in which US nurses and other health professionals are educated and practice.

The first challenge, according to the Pew Health Professions Commission report, is to *redesign* the ways in which health professional work is organised. All settings must be included in the redesign process – hospitals, private offices, clinics, community practices and public health. Health professional education, as it currently exists, produces practitioners who are very cost-intensive. This means that nurses, physicians and other allied health professionals must continually justify their cost (in terms of compensation, benefits and continuing education requirements) by expanding their realm of practice and influence to needy clients beyond their own geographical confines.

Using innovative approaches such as telecommunications technology, practitioners can devise telehealth initiatives that greatly expand their expertise and practice. This can be accomplished through long-distance specialist consultation with colleagues in remote sites; patient education on-line for clients living with chronic illness and disability, or elderly individuals who need clear, repeated self-care encouragement and instructions; and remote practice itself, where X-ray and laboratory results can be analysed at a central location and quickly interpreted for clients at the other end. In the future, none of us will be able to say, 'I can only be in one place at a time'.

The second challenge is to *reregulate* the ways in which health professionals are permitted to practise, allowing more flexibility and experimentation. Licensing and certification (now under the authority of the individual state in which the professional practises) must, particularly with the expansion of telecommunications capacity, be simplified and standardised for those who will practise in a number of states simultaneously.

Right-sizing the health professional workforce and the institutions that produce health professionals is imperative. The Pew Commission report makes specific recommendations for closing schools of medicine and nursing to halt overproduction. Federal and state subsidies for education that are tied to care delivery must be broken. Included in US Medicare reform proposals are provisions to reduce the current $13 billion Graduate Medical Education Fund, which is used to subsidise physician clinical residency slots in teaching hospitals. (Some nursing programmes have also benefited from these funds.) Any future subsidy must relate directly to the workforce needs of the country. The nursing community is hoping to garner some of these monies to support the training of advanced practice nurses in primary care. Present-day health workforce needs are for more primary care practitioners (family physicians, paediatricians, nurse midwives and nurse practitioners) and fewer specialty care professionals.

Last, the report makes recommendations for the *restructuring* of education for health professionals. Accountability, in terms of cost, consumer satisfaction and positive outcomes, is the pervasive watch-word in the health industry today, and educational institutions can no longer escape its imperative. Schools have in the past produced practitioners with the skills that they wanted to supply. In the future, institutions that can respond to the demands of the emerging health care system will be favoured. This will translate into changes in the skills, competences, and knowledge base of all health professions, including the process by which education is regulated, the length of education and the costs of education. Accreditation and licensing processes must be looked at anew, with an eye towards increased public governance. Traditional accreditation procedures have been an impediment to change because educational institutions have, in their quest to maintain accreditation, been denied the flexibility needed to respond to innovation, social need and demand (Pew Health Professions Commission, 1995).

NURSING POLICY RESPONSE TO CURRENT TRENDS IN US HEALTH POLICY

The phenomenal developments in health policy just described have greatly influenced the ways in which the USA thinks about its health, how it receives care, how it funds the health care system and how individuals regard their own well-being, quality of life and responsibility for maintaining it. Other factors that help to shape and form US health care policy are gleaned from comparisons with the international community. Key issues in evaluating and comparing health care systems are access to care, the level of health expenditure, public satisfaction with health care, and the overall quality of care as expressed by the health of the population (Bodenheimer and Grumbach, 1995).

In a 1990 survey of 10 nations conducted by Robert Blendon at the Harvard School of Public Health, Canada ranked first in public satis-faction with its health care system, Germany ranked third, the UK eighth, and the USA came in last (Blendon *et al.*, 1990). Comparisons of health care quality are difficult to make and can only convey gross comparisons, but the fact that the USA has an infant mortality rate higher than that of Germany, Canada and the UK is indicative of the fact that the American health care system does not work well in all areas. In terms of life expectancy, another gross indicator of quality of health care, Canada has the highest male and female life expectancy rates at birth. The life expectancy rate at age 80 ranks highest in Canada and the USA compared with Germany and the UK. The life expectancy rate at age 80 is more a measure of the impact of health care, especially its high-technology component.

Health expenditure comparisons show the USA paying the highest per capita amount and the highest total health expenditures as a percentage of gross domestic product (Table 2.3). It should also be noted that between 35 and 40 million people in the USA have no health insurance coverage, which often translates into little or no access to the health care system. The debate over whether health care is a right or a privilege still rages on across the Atlantic, and recent proposals in the 103rd Congress that would have provided universal access to care failed to pass despite strong support from President Clinton and many concerned Americans, including nurses.

Table 2.3   Total health expenditures as a percentage of gross domestic product, 1960–95

	1960	1970	1980	1990	1995
Germany	4.7	5.5	7.9	8.3	10.4
United Kingdom	3.9	4.5	5.8	6.2	6.9
Canada	5.5	7.2	7.4	9.5	9.6
United States	5.2	7.4	9.2	12.2	14.2

Source: OECD, 1997

Nursing policy for the 21st century is a product of both the internal events described previously and an external comparison with our global partners. In addition, the vision of professional nurses committed to care continually shapes and moulds the process. Components of the emerging US health care system can serve as a compass to steer the formulation of future policy. These include:

● increasing reliance on primary care, health promotion and disease prevention

- continuous quality improvement in the delivery of care, including the move towards evidence-based practice
- a lowering of the overall cost of health care by producing practitioners who meet societal need and demand
- enhancing patient satisfaction and consumer involvement in health care.

Policy for nursing education will need to prepare nurses who can readily take up health policy trends and chart an appropriate course for practice and research. Characteristics that are salient to education and the clinical preparation of nurses in the next century are curricula that orientate student nurses toward health very early in their educational experience, population-based perspectives that provide the opportunity to develop competence in working with culturally diverse communities and conducting basic public health epidemiological assessments. Nurses are in an ideal position to guide and direct communities toward optimal health through school-based clinics, community centres, ambulatory care facilities and home health settings.

Additional areas of curriculum change include:

- training in the intensive use and understanding of information and telecommunications technology
- developing an approach to clients and treatment outcomes that are consumer centred
- client management competences that successfully help clients to make care transitions from one setting to another
- a keen respect for accountability as the true hallmark of professional nursing practice
- opportunities that foster interdependent practice and a multidisciplinary team approach to client care (Pew Health Professions Commission, 1995).

These areas are policy imperatives as well as sound building blocks for the growth of a nursing profession well poised to make a substantial contribution to the future of health care.

The real challenge for American nurses comes when they try to transform their knowledge about achieving successful outcomes for their clients, along with the professional beliefs that they hold for the future of health care delivery, into a national policy for health. It takes tremendous political will to shape an entire system because, ultimately, it is a political act. As America's collective value system is committed to low taxes, pluralism and entrepreneurialism, politicians and policy-makers have been unsuccessful in their attempts to craft a more equitable health care system. Fortunately, nursing policy has always benefited from a strong political base fuelled and energised by nurses all across the USA. Every major group representing nurses sends lobbyists to Washington to advocate for and propose policy that meets nursing's agenda for our nation's health and well-being. Nurses, back in their respective home states, have come together to form a powerful and effective grass-roots lobbying network. This effort facilitates the work of nursing leaders in Washington. Money is donated to candidates who are supportive of nursing's agenda and has, in some instances, aided in the election of nurse legislators at the state and federal level. Maryland, for example, currently has five nurse legislators serving in the General Assembly in Annapolis, making a substantial difference to the kind and quality of health legislation that is debated and eventually passed into law.

Nursing's policy interests cover a broad array of issues and concerns, including:

- the federal subsidisation of nurse education programmes
- direct reimbursement for advanced practice nurses
- prescriptive privileges and authority for independent practice at the state level
- the extension of primary care services to underserved areas
- curbing the overemphasis on cost in the largely unregulated managed care industry
- pursuing the inclusion of antidiscrimination language in every major health care reform proposal, language that prevents non-physician providers being denied access to managed care networks
- advocating for equitable Medicare, Medicaid and welfare reform.

In closing, let us re-emphasise that the most critical challenge for US nursing in the future is the longer-term transition to fully inte-grated delivery systems in which competition for capitation contracts will be great (Buerhaus, 1996). All health care organisa-tions must be encouraged to compete on the basis of not only cost, but also quality. Implementing a quality agenda will serve the profession of nursing well. Ensuring value means focusing on cost and quality as one and the same variable. This will separate health provider survivors from those who either simply cease to exist or are replaced by more cost-effective alternatives. Strong management skills will be essential to nurses' future viability as providers under financial arrangements where all in the health care market face identical incentives.

Nurses, through education, practice, and research, will need to be able to operationalise wellness, prevention and primary care effectively. These will be the glue that holds the emerging health system together (Buerhaus, 1996). Illness prevention and wellness will replace costly disease models of care. Every provider faced with cost constraints and capitation reimbursement will be financially motivated to provide only the care required. Here, the practice perspective of nurses can make a notable difference. Advanced practice nurses, in particular, can provide services that are 'value added', which means that cost, quality, positive client outcomes and consumer satisfaction are addressed within a context of holistic, culturally appropriate care.

Health trends and evolving health policy have and will continue to have an enormous impact on the education and practice of nurses in the USA. Similarly, nursing innovation, stimulated by research, will exert a tremendous influence on patterns of care, consumer participation and satisfaction, and the design of service delivery models. The relationship between health policy and nursing policy is reciprocal and mutually reinforcing; herein lies the greatest hope for the future of health care and the future of nursing in the USA.

REFERENCES

Blendon, R.J. Benson, J. and Donelan, C. (1990) Satisfaction with health systems in ten nations. *Health Affairs* **9**(2): 185.

Bodenheimer, T.S. and Grumbach, K. (1995) *Understanding Health Policy: A Clinical Approach*. Norwalk, CO: Appleton & Lange.

Buerhaus. P.I. (1996) Quality and cost: the value of consumer and nurse partnerships. *Nursing Policy Forum*: 12–20.

Hurst, J.W. (1991) Reforming health care in seven European nations. *Health Affairs* **10**(3): 7–21.

Iglehart, J.K. (1991) Editorial. *Health Affairs* **10**(3): 5–6.

Marmour, T. and Oberlander, J. (1998) Rethinking medicine reform. *Health Affairs* **17**(1), Jan–Feb.

Pew Health Professions Commission (1995) *Critical Challenges: Revitalising the Health Care Professions for the Twenty First Century*. Third Report of the Pew Health Professions Commission. San Francisco: UCSF Center for the Health Professions.

Organisation for Economic Cooperation and Development (1997) *Health Data 97*. Paris: OECD.

CHAPTER THREE

Nurses' influence on health policy in Australia

Sandra C. Legg and Sonia J. Zyntek

Editors' Introduction

This chapter discusses six policy areas that Australian nurses have influenced: nurse education; case mix funding and case management; industrial relations; remote area nursing and aboriginal health; the beginnings of the euthanasia debate; and ecology. Nurses' involvement in the six policy processes has been varied. An example of strong professional leadership is described in the section on industrial relations, and a visionary nurse leader is described who influenced the introduction of education and registration of aboriginal health workers to serve their own populations. The latter is an example of a problem – limited health care in aboriginal communities – that was raised to the political agenda and led to the formation of a policy to alleviate the situation. Networking and pressure groups are highlighted in the discussion on ecology.

INTRODUCTION

The global position and national geography of Australia, as well as the demographics of its people, have been a major driving force behind the significant contribution that Australian nurses have made to the development and implementation of policy in health care.

Although a large country, Australia has a relatively small population of approximately 18 million people. This equates to a population density of two persons per square kilometre of surface area, compared with 326 people per square kilometre in Japan, 234 in the UK, and 102 in France.

The majority of people live in large coastal urban and suburban areas, but many occupy rural and isolated communities. Much of central Australia is desert. Providing equitable services, in particular health care services, to communities that are so diverse, both in location and population, is not feasible. The greater suburban and urban communities benefit from a well-resourced health care system with a wide choice of specialised and highly skilled health care professionals, easily accessible and well-equipped facilities and all the advantages of modern technology. Although rural and isolated communities have access to a range of health care resources, their location limits resource availability and they do not have the same ease of access to the major services and technologies enjoyed by their counterparts in suburban and urban Australia.

In the isolated areas of Australia, there are 200 locations where health care is provided wholly by nurses who consult with doctors by radio. In less isolated rural areas where there is a doctor, she or he may practise in two or more towns or districts, so nurses still have the major responsibility for health care.

The Australian health care system can be characterised as a mixed system in the way in which it is financed and organised. The public sector is the dominant component, hospitals being funded and managed by government. There is, however, a small and proactive private hospital and private health insurance industry. The medical profession, operating on a fee-for-service basis, is very influential and political.

While the federal government, through Medicare (the national health insurance scheme), subsidises medical services directly, it provides funds to the states for the operation of the public health care system. Australia's cost containment strategy has consisted of three key elements: the control of hospital budgets at a state level, the control of capital expenditure at the state level, and physician fee controls by the federal government. All Australian states have moved to decentralised management for the public system, and to global budgets for financial controls.

Unlike the UK, area health authorities and purchaser/provider arrangements have not been implemented to date, although this is currently under review. Case mix funding has, however, been introduced into the public hospital system and to a lesser extent into the private system.

Australia is currently pursuing a rigorous approach to policy, and its influence exists in several key areas:

- the consumers' participation in health reform
- research and health policy development

- qualitative and quantitative approaches to evaluation in health care
- mental health reform
- a national aboriginal health strategy
- a national food and safety policy
- policy determinants in rehabilitation
- evaluating medical technology
- Australia's international health relations.

Australia shares with other technologically advanced societies the two-edged consequences of its own medical successes. While Australians enjoy better health, a serious incompatibility exists between what is now technically possible, the access to health services and the limit put on health care spending. Within this environment of economic rationing, nurses have challenged some of the dominant interests in the health sector, to the advancement of the profession and national health care services.

Australian nursing in the 1980s made huge gains in the interconnected areas of education, professionalisation, political visibility and improvements in pay and conditions. In the 1990s, nurses sustained this political activity and effectiveness while at the same time adopting a whole new language, new strategies and new aims. Among their many achievements, Australian nurses have had significant influence in shaping policies for:

- nurse education
- case mix funding and case management
- industrial relations
- remote area nursing and aboriginal health
- the beginnings of the euthanasia debate
- discovering an ecological self.

POLICY ACHIEVEMENTS

The impact of tertiary education

Professional nursing in Australia has travelled a long, often challenging and demanding road since its beginnings in 1868 when six nurses trained in the Nightingale system arrived in Sydney. The Nightingale system of apprenticeship training remained relatively unchanged for over 100 years. It met Australia's need for a rapidly growing workforce to staff the increasing number of hospitals throughout the country and was significant in the establishment of nursing as a profession.

Over the past three decades, the roles, responsibilities and expectations of nurses have changed significantly in Australia, culminating in a dramatic change in the way in which nurses are educated. Pressure for this change has come from many quarters, for example:

- continuous strong criticism of the apprenticeship system; for example, clinical learning experiences were unstructured, student nurses were poorly paid (cheap labour) and overregulated, and the apprenticeship approach of 'learning by doing' was incompatible with government and community attitudes to education
- in what is predominantly a female profession, women's altered work expectations (secondary to the women's movement in the 1970s)
- the strong belief, supported by numerous reports, that the standard of nursing education must be raised and the education system for nurses therefore changed.
- the recognition that it was not only essential, but also that nurses had a right, to receive education that was based on and encouraged critical thinking and the development of individual potential
- the need for nursing to keep abreast of the changing knowledge and technologies in the medical field and how they related to nursing practice
- the necessity for multiskilling and greater efficiency and productivity in the face of economic pressures.

In 1984 the Commonwealth government of the day decided that nurse education should be totally transferred to the higher education sector. Nine years later, in 1993, the transfer was completed. For many, the move to tertiary education heralded the initial preparation for lifelong professional practice and learning. Tertiary education differed dramatically from the apprenticeship style of training in that it brought with it better resources, higher standards, a broader knowledge base and a greater element of self-management in learning.

Nurses who have qualified in the tertiary system recognise and embrace the opportunities now available to them. There is a continuing and increasing demand for places in the 34 Australian universities with faculties or schools of nursing for undergraduate degrees and related graduate diplomas, higher degrees and more recently doctorates (available in about half of the schools of nursing).

One of the more recent and significant growth areas in nursing is that of research. Universities have made a major contribution not only to nurses' acquisition of knowledge and skills in research methodology, but also in stimulating research-based practice and the promotion of research in applied clinical nursing. The further development and continuation of this trend is vital to the future of nursing, the expanding role of the nurse and the continued provision of evidence-based practice.

The graduate nurse of the 1990s in Australia will be prepared to face the growing and changing health care challenges of the new millennium with confidence, accountability and direction, contributing to and building on expanding areas of research to ensure that the health care needs of all Australians are met.

Case mix and case management

Case mix, defined as the classification and costing of patients within a DRG, together with case management, defined as the management of a patient's total episode of care from preadmission to discharge home, were introduced into the Australian health care system in 1994. Since then, a number of developments have taken place on all aspects of case mix. For example, the DRG classification has been modified by Australian health professionals to suit their circumstances. Other case mix systems are being adopted or designed to cover subacute inpatient, ambulatory and other forms of care, and most recently a system for costing home care. Clinical indicators are being developed to improve measurement and control of care, and several experiments in clinical resource management are under way. Prudent costing systems used throughout the public health system have recently been introduced into the private system. The private sector had previously been funded on length of stay, rather than on episodic payments.

Senior nurse leaders in New South Wales have been at the forefront of leading the national agenda and have jointly chaired the national working party for case mix implementation. Australian nurses are determined to help to set the case mix agenda in order to ensure maximum quality outcomes for patients. Most of the public health system now has several projects in both acute and community care and some are in the process of evaluation. The impact that case mix methodologies may have on nursing care is still not clearly defined, but Australian nurses are working hard to find solutions from the evaluations already undertaken. The first challenge for nurses over the next decade, however, will be to set standards of clinical practice such as the over- or underuse of services, the wrong location or the improper use of services. Setting standards in respect of outcomes measures is therefore critical to the future development of quality care.

Australian nurses have similarly been very proactive in leading the case management and critical pathways agenda, again leading government national working parties and guiding policy at the highest political levels. This is viewed in contrast to the situation in the UK where other disciplines, such as professions allied to medicine and business managers, are often in the driving seat.

It can be seen from this that Australian nurse leaders have really taken the initiative in leading a national health care strategy. In taking the lead, they have undoubtedly empowered knowledgeable nurse managers, and nursing in general, to be at the forefront of a government-prioritised health care issue.

Industrial relations

Trade unionism in Australia has had a turbulent and rocky path. The rise and power of the Australian Nurses Federation (ANF) in the 1980s and 90s demonstrated a more consistent approach to nursing and industrial relations issues. Prior to the 1980s, Australian nurses were a docile group of workers, and employers were vigorously opposed to the ANF's claims for better conditions. However, over the past two decades, nurses have become more assertive and increasingly successful in making industrial gains. Nurses in New South Wales serve as an obvious example of the positive change in nurses' attitudes to industrial relations. The New South Wales Nurses Association (NSWNA), a state branch of the ANF, has achieved and maintained a healthy membership. Although nurses continue to join the NSWNA for practical rather than ideological reasons, they now accept that trade unionism is a legitimate means of protecting and advancing their interests. In 1992, the NSWNA was described as 'Australia's best trade union'.

With a change in leadership in 1987 and working under the slogan of 'Nurses for Unity', the NSWNA set their sights on professional pay rates for nurses that took account of the shift to tertiary qualifications for registered nurses. Wage rates improved at a faster rate than wages generally in the community. Moreover, the position of registered nurses improved compared with that of other Australian women. Thus, by the late 1980s, the NSWNA was bargaining from a position of strength even though Australia's general economic climate was poor and the government was seeking to cut health costs and reduce services.

Every opportunity for public meetings, conferences and the use of Sky Television for industrial as well as educational purposes was used, and in latter years the NSWNA's image with both public and private employers has been that of a numerically strong union with a direct and aggressive style of industrial negotiation.

As a result of strong leadership that fostered positive industrial growth, the nursing profession stands united in fighting for human rights, justice, the ethics of health care, patients' rights and the empowerment of nursing staff. Nurse executives and nurse academics in New South Wales have grown in knowledge and understanding of legal and industrial issues. They are a mature group of leaders who have set the course of nursing history in New South Wales, and more widely in Australia, by bringing a large workforce behind them in solidarity and commitment.

Remote area nursing and aboriginal health

Remote area nurses (RANs) are working in remote areas all over Australia and its territories, with a concentrated population in the northern tropical zone and central and western desert areas of Western Australia, Queensland, Torres Strait Islands and the Northern Territory. They are employed by state and territory health departments, independent aboriginal health services and church-affiliated organisations.

A recent study by Cramer (1995) indicated that out of 33 remote communities, 42.5 per cent had a one-nurse post and 30.5 per cent a two-nurse post. In 27 per cent of the other communities, there were three, four or five nurses. The populations of these remote communities ranged from 250 to more than 2,000. Most nurses work in remote aboriginal communities where indigenous languages are spoken. In addition, RANs travel to conduct clinics in outstations on a weekly basis. The majority of them work in communities that are located between 400 and 2,500 km from their administrative centres. The majority of RANs rely on the Royal Flying Doctor Services or the Aerial Medical Service for the emergency evacuation of patients to regional hospital bases. In some cases, nurses transport patients themselves, either in 'half-way meets' with a road ambulance service or to a regional hospital.

In each Australian state, there are health policies specifically for Aborigines, who make up 1 per cent of the population. Nurses are at the forefront of policy development for aboriginal health, in particular through the ANF and the Royal College of Nursing Australia (RCNA). Both associations were influential in the publication of an Aboriginal and Torres Strait Islanders Affairs Strategy, focusing on aboriginal health, which continues to languish at levels comparable with those of the most underdeveloped of Third World Countries. The average life expectancy at birth for Aborigines is still 15–20 years less than for other Australians.

The National Aboriginal Health Strategy published in 1989 has recently been evaluated by the ANF, and its findings have stimulated change in a number of areas and practical fields that are not working. A recent conference for remote area nurses has set a future strategy for dealing with these deficits, with recommendations to the federal minister of health.

A major influence in aboriginal health has been the introduction of the aboriginal health worker. Aboriginal health workers are members of the local community and are selected by the community health council to be health workers. The workers are always responsible for their community, and although an 'on-call' system operates when there is an emergency, the health workers are expected to adopt the responsible caring role.

It was Ellen Kettle, a remote area nurse/tutor of distinction, now retired, who influenced the education and registration of aboriginal health workers. In Australia, there are no full-blooded aboriginal registered or enrolled nurses, since aboriginals only manage about 6 or 7 years of school education and this therefore prevents their access to nursing faculties of education. Kettle recognised how essential it was for a group of aboriginals to be trained in health issues in order to serve and influence their own community health standards. Aboriginal health workers have a modular programme and courses catering for illiteracy. Today, influenced and driven by nurses, there is a national system for the education and registration of aboriginal health workers. Hennessy (1988), on her National Florence Nightingale Scholarship to Australia, recommended that many lessons can be learned from this programme for dealing with the health and well-being of indigenous peoples of any culture.

Ethical and reflective practice

In September 1997, a man from Darwin in the Northern Territory became the first person to die under the new Northern Territory's euthanasia legislation. At that time, at least five other Australians were waiting to die under the rights of the Terminally Ill Act. Bob Dent, aged 66, a former carpenter and pilot, died after using a computer-linked machine that administered lethal drugs. He had suffered prostate cancer for 5 years.

The news of Bob Dent's death prompted a heated debate around the nation, with expressions of outrage from church leaders and divisions among politicians over a proposal before federal parliament to over-turn the Northern Territory law. In an open letter to federal parliamen-tarians, Bob Dent said: 'If you disagree with voluntary euthanasia, then don't use it, but don't deny me the right to use it if and when I want to' (*The Age*, 27 September 1996).

In recognition of the significance of changing social attitudes towards the ethics of life and death, and the potential impact of these changes on the profession and the practice of nursing, the RCNA has canvassed views from the nursing profession on the issue of euthanasia. In the light of the diversity of views, the RCNA has issued a number of guidelines (1996), including an RCNA position paper on euthanasia.

The International Council of Nurses (ICN) *Code for Nurses* (1973) indicates that the fundamental responsibilities of nurses are to promote health, prevent illness, restore health and alleviate suffering. These concepts are reflected in all the Australian codes for nurses, including the Code of Ethics for Nurses in Australia (ANCI, 1993). This code, however, argues 'No' in response to the question 'Does the nurse's responsibility to alleviate suffering extend to assisting the patient to die, or even to kill the patient, in an act of voluntary euthanasia?'

Australian nurses are demonstrating a strong clear voice in the ethical arena and are already voicing their position in the euthanasia debate. Academics such as Johnstone (1989) continue to guide poli-cies and advise the government. Her work and thinking is 'Australia-made' but is also 'export quality'. Johnstone has contributed a great deal to the moral/ethical debate in nursing and is at the forefront of influencing the euthanasia debate for the future.

Nurses in Australia today are being encouraged to ensure that the practical problem-solving domains of practice are not given prece-dence over the domains of ethical and reflective practice. Small (1996, p. 60) develops this further when she emphasises that the 'ethical pattern of knowing forms the basis of reflective practice which has the potential for facilitating nurses' decision making, as they question and critically analyse their everyday practice'. Nurses swept up in the euthanasia debate, who are struggling to maintain patient-centred care and similarly deal with the technological revolution, must, as Small emphasises, continue to move beyond the more restrictive empirical ways of knowing to a more ethical pattern of knowing. This ethical pattern of knowing where euthanasia is concerned is, at the moment, firmly monitored by the *Code of Ethics for Nurses in Australia* (ACNI, 1993). This does not mean to say, however, that ethical academic pursuit cannot change the sands of time for the future.

The ecological self in Australian nursing

The ecological self in Australian nursing explores the notion that nurses are developing their political will as a natural extension of advocacy for their patients and the communities they serve, while at the same time developing a deep ecological self (Lacroix, 1996). Naess (1986) referred to the ecological self as an 'ultimate form of self-realisation' that is widened and deepened as we see ourselves in nature. According to Lacroix (1996, p. 9), 'ecological selfhood in nursing is therefore a two way process which reinforces the notion that: care of the self and patients/clients is care of the natural environment, care of the environment is care of the self and patients/clients'.

This concept of an ecological self is beautifully described by Vicky Walker in her address on aboriginal spirituality, at the first National Health and Ecology Conference:

> People can't still understand why they have no relationship, no sitting on the land and experiencing the life that's in the land. Life is there in the land, it talks to you, it's there. And you hear the animals, the little insects, the birds, the rivers flowing wherever you are. But you need to take time. Where I come from, Lake Mungo, when I walk on the earth its like I have not feet. It's like my feet are down in the earth and there's nothing between me and the earth. You can feel that your being is coming from that land and you can feel your ancestors' presence. And that too gives you energy. So it's all those factors that make us, that helped us live and survive all this time. (Walker, 1993, p. 194)

The notion of ecological selfhood developed by Australian nurses, of our dependence on the natural environment for human health and survival, is now affirmed by scientists and the nursing profession. The Union of Concerned Scientists published an urgent warning to humanity, calling for 'the stewardship of the earth in order to avoid total environmental degradation' (Lacroix, 1996, p. 11). Nursing visionaries from all over Australia are now highly vocal in their declaration for a nursing commitment to the natural environment and the planet. The ANF's value statement reinforces the notion of an ecological ethic of care. Value Statement number 6 affirms that:

> Nurses value the promotion of an ecological, social and economic environment which supports and sustains health and well-being.

In 1993, eight nurses active in environmental issues in nursing were invited to participate in a qualitative multiple case study. The participants reflected upon five basic questions on the future of nursing and ecological sustainability. Ecological attributes identified through this process were (as cited in Lacroix, 1996):

1. *connectedness*: having a fundamental connectedness between a healthy self, a healthy community and a healthy natural environment
2. *reciprocity*: being receptive, open and sensitive to the teachings and wisdom of the natural environment
3. *simplicity*: having a singleness of purpose, sincerity and honesty within, as well as avoidance of clutter and possessions.

Scientific writers, thinkers and philosophers suggest that the largest challenges facing the scientific and professional communities today are large-scale environmental degradation, such as climatic change, depletion of the ozone layer, acid rain and land degradation. Climatic change alone, according to the National Health and Medical Research Council (1991), could result in an increased risk of skin cancer, eye damage, respiratory symptoms, water-borne diseases, heat stress and vector-borne disease. Even more difficult to predict are the potential effects that environmental degradation has on the social well-being of communities.

There is therefore no doubt that the health of the population is intrinsically related to the health of the environment. Nursing is in a unique position to influence ecological policies and should draw on Nightingale's skills as a social reformer, statistician, hygienist and political manipulator, all of which make her an appropriate role model for the profession as it strives to refocus on ecological public health.

Australian nurses have recognised the authenticity of the many concerns addressed by environmental groups, scientists and philosophers, and have formed many groups to address prevention and remediation at local level. Bogossian (1996), however, in concert with her colleagues in Lacroix (1996), emphasises the fact that nursing's ability to respond to ecological concern depends on its ability to think and develop ways of knowing that extend beyond traditional environmental boundaries. She challenges the profession in its ability to think and to develop new ways of *knowing* in order to extend its professional scope of practice toward the development of an ecological self in nursing.

Changes in the workplace can be brought about in a variety of ways, one very effective way being that of participatory action research that is directed at ecological sustainability. Street (1996) references the EcoHealth Project in a Melbourne hospital, conducted by Helen Lucas (Lucas, 1996). The main focus of this study was on waste management. Key to the success of this project was the involvement of all possible stakeholders. These people were formed into ecological health communities who worked on a problem-solving model with inbuilt evaluation and reflective processes at the completion of each action strategy.

In the EcoHealth study, each ecological health community identified its common concerns and researchable issues which included the following (Street, 1996, pp. 91–2):

- The identification of infectious and non-infectious waste, to develop proper segregation and examine the issues for clinical practice in a cardiac-thoracic unit.
- An orthopaedic ward was concerned about the high usage of the disposable continence care sheets.
- The operating room had a number of sound ecological practices in place and decided that a staff education programme was required to keep the momentum going.
- The medical research laboratory was concerned about the pouring of solvents down the sinks.
- The waste management committee wanted to change its structure and focus to involve sub-committees of activists to achieve some changes in the hospital.

Some hospital nurses, however, have little opportunity for appreciating the whole contextual nature of the patient, and Parker (1993, p. 89) argues that nurses need to 'be able to cross disciplinary boundaries, to communicate in plain language and to work collaboratively with others in addressing the health issues that face us globally and in our day to day work situations'.

Current trends in the health system, such as managed care, early discharge and case mix funding, offer many opportunities for emphasising the notion that the home is a healing environment. Hoare (1996, p. 74) stresses that, with a focus on community care, the challenge for nurses will be to demonstrate the effectiveness of care with an ecological focus. The challenge for educators will be to provide a curriculum that is broadly based and highlights the relationship between lifestyle and human and planetary health. Finally, Hoare (1996, p. 75) predicts that Australian nurses are on the road to moving from and beyond the confines of care of the person, to care of the household, the community and the planet.

THE GOLD RUSH FOR OWNERSHIP

Australia in the 1880s saw a great rush for gold in the newly discovered goldfields of the country, and at the height of gold rush mania, it seemed as though some new and 'foreign' group of gold-diggers was staking a claim in the 'race for gold' almost every day. Similarly, in the 1990s, a rush is on for staking claims and holding ownership in the development and implementation of health policies. An incessant hoopla over the rationalisation of services and who is doing what has created a gold rush atmosphere, which is predicted to continue for some time.

With certain assumptions predicted for the millennium and beyond, nurses must position themselves carefully within this gold rush atmosphere. These assumptions include advances in science and technology, an extended life expectancy, alternative modalities of living, expanding world economies with enhanced opportunities for sharing health promotion internationally and burgeoning information and rapid transit systems.

Based on these future assumptions, nurses will be uniquely placed to adopt a whole new language for influencing change and the development of health policy. There are many opportunities: the shift in the roles of doctors and nurses; the focus on primary care and health promotion; the development of the operating room registered nurse First Assistant and the independent nurse practitioner; nursing expertise in case mix and case management; the commitment to best practice, standards and competences; the consumer-orientated society; the dominance of ethical and reflective practice; and the necessity for an ecologically sustainable future.

CONCLUSION

The critical path for Australian nurses as they move towards the millennium has been one of political action, educational revival, corporate bonding and the growth of nursing knowledge. Within the economic rationalisation of the Australian health system, nurses have encountered many challenging and unprecedented health care issues. They can be justly proud of their achievements thus far and can be congratulated on their political ability and know-how, as well as perhaps on being, on occasions, in the right place at the right time. Certain factors have been in their favour:

- Australia is a federation of states. This enables empowerment and decision-making at a more local level of the service and 'frees up' the nursing profession's structure and constitutional arrangements.
- Australia has had a massive immigration policy over the last 50 years, and this has presented a challenge in developing and sharing skills in a new and creative way.
- Australia was founded by 'tough' pioneers who worked under incredibly hard environmental conditions. Australian women, therefore, have inherited a pioneering spirit, which is evident in the nursing profession's strategies for breaking 'new ground' and for risk-taking ventures.
- The Australian federal government's commitment to tertiary education has instilled a certain confidence in the profession's ability to 'stand tall', and 9 years of nursing education taking place in universities have enabled nurses to contribute to policy in an academic and critical way.

There are some extraordinarily talented people in the nursing profession who will contribute to new visions of what the profession can achieve. If nursing can combine its expertise and talents, and keep listening to patients, it has a chance of leading the way and impacting health policy for the future. The dawn of the communication revolution, creating a learning environment and being smart, offers the profession every opportunity. Nurses must sustain the impact they have already achieved on policy to prepare for the future demands and ethical dilemmas that lie ahead.

REFERENCES

Australian Nursing Council Incorporated (1993) *Code of Ethics for Nurses in Australia.* Developed by ANCI, RCNA & ANF. Canberra: ANCI.

Bogossian, F. (1996) Empiricism, environmentalism and ecological public health. In Lacroix, D. (ed.) *The Ecological Self in Australian Nursing.* Canberra: Royal College of Nursing, Australia.

Cramer, J. (1995) Finding solutions to support remote area nurses. *Australian Nursing Journal* (Dec/Jan): **2**(6).

Hennessy, D.A. (1988) *The Organisation of Health Care and Nursing Education in Israel and Australia.* National Florence Nightingale Scholarship Report. Lodged in the Royal College of Nursing Library, London.

Hoare, T. (1996) A deep ecology of community nursing. In Lacroix, D. (ed.) *The Ecological Self in Australian Nursing.* Canberra: Royal College of Nursing, Australia.

International Council of Nurses (1973) *Code for Nurses: Ethical Concepts Applied to Nursing.* Geneva: ICN.

Johnstone, M.-J. (1989) *Bioethics: A Nursing Perspective.* Sydney: Harcourt Brace Jovanovich.

Lacroix, D. (1996) Awakening an ecological self. In Lacroix, D. (ed.) *The Ecological Self in Australian Nursing.* Canberra: Royal College of Nursing, Australia.

Lucas, H. (1996) Personal communications. In Lacroix, D. (ed.) *The Ecological Self in Australian Nursing.* Canberra: Royal College of Nursing, Australia.

Naess, A. (1986) Self-realisation: an ecological approach to being in the world. In Van De Veer, D. and Pierce, C. (eds) *The Environmental Ethics and Policy Book. Philosophy, Ecology, Economics.* California: Wadsworth.

National Health and Medical Research Council (1991) *Ecologically Sustainable Development: The Health Perspective.* Canberra: AGPS.

Parker, J. (1993) Toward a nursing ethic for sustainable planetary health. In *Health and Ecology: A Nursing Perspective,* pp. 87–92. Conference proceedings, March.

Royal College of Nursing Australia (1996) Booklet of resources to accompany the Video: *Rights of the Terminally Ill Act: Nurses and Voluntary Euthanasia.* Canberra: Royal College of Nursing, Australia.

Small, J. (1996) Ethical knowing through ecological awareness. In Lacroix , D. (ed.) *The Ecological Self in Australian Nursing.* Australia: Royal College of Nursing, Australia.

Street, A. (1996) Ecological thinking through the action research process. In Lacroix, D. (ed.) *The Ecological Self in Australian Nursing.* Canberra: Royal College of Nursing, Australia.

Union of Concerned Scientists (1992) Press Release: *World's Leading Scientists Issue Urgent Warning to Humanity,* Washington, DC.

Walker, V. (1993) Aboriginal spirituality. In Newman, N. (ed.) *Health and Ecology: A Nursing Perspective.* Proceedings of First National Conference, Nursing the Environment. Melbourne: Australian Nurses Federation.

Nursing policy – strategic approaches

An international perspective

Trevor J. Ride

Editors' Introduction

This chapter complements the first chapter by concentrating more on nursing policy itself. It will be noted that the definition of policy in this chapter is slightly different from that provided in Chapter 1. This does not mean that one is incorrect but instead serves to illustrate the lack of clarity surrounding the terms used and emphasises how important it is to try to understand how a term is employed in any situation and how others understand it. The text provides an interesting debate on the interaction between strategy and policy. The focus is on nursing policy globally. The author, having defined nursing policy, describes how nurses are using the three elements of nursing policy originally described by Nightingale to contribute to the changing global health need. The specificity as well as the differentiation across the world health sector is emphasised.

INTRODUCTION – THE BASIS OF POLICY

Policy is not a complex subject in itself, but there is much written on the subject that makes it appear so. The perspective taken in this chapter is that policy is about problem-solving and developing solutions. The complexity comes from the context, the environment and knowledge of the situations for which solutions are sought or policy is being developed. Developing problem-solving skills is part of the developmental learning process. Extending this into the area of policy concerns transferring the framework and skills of problem-solving from everyday life to this specific subject area.

The questions relating to policy in any sphere cannot be considered in isolation but need to relate to the context, setting and culture of where the question is posed and what is actually meant (Mintzberg and Quinn, 1991). There is such a vast and complex literature on the subjects of policy, strategy and related matters that the reader can become confused over what is meant or indeed what is being referred to. A useful perspective of policy is to consider the extent to which it relates to approaches in problem-solving, change situations and solutions. The fundamental questions present themselves as:

- What is policy?
- What do we mean by it?
- Why do we have it?

Some sources link the term 'policy' with that of strategy and use them both synonymously, while others differentiate between them (Mintzberg, 1994). In the organisational context, the terms are also used in ways relevant to the setting or organisation (or even the levels within an organisation) in which they are being used. It is common to come across organisations in both the public and private sector, as well as at national and local levels, that use language such as 'strategic direction', 'organisational strategy' and 'operational strategy' to mean either the same or quite different things. Whether or not there is any real difference has now become a matter of general semantics. Some organisations will develop a strategic direction and organisational policies for the same activities albeit under a different name.

Even if the literature on policy does not help the understanding of the nature of policy (or strategy), there is a difference as described in dictionary definitions (for example, *Concise Oxford Dictionary*):

Strategic = serving the ends, plan formed according to policy
Policy   = plan for action

Implicit in strategy is some sense of vision, purpose or aim and forming plans underpinned by values. Quite specifically, policy is described more clearly in terms of plans for action. What must be stressed is that none of these terms is absolute, and if it is employed as such, its use is dependent upon time, place, setting and other variables. There must be a common understanding in terms of what is actually meant by this variety of terms. In essence, strategy and policy become a concept, and addressing and considering this concept can help the understanding of policy, its development and its analysis.

In addition to vision, strategy is quite commonly (although not exclusively) used to describe and define scenario, direction or, put simply, some kind of future and outcome underpinned by values. It could be suggested that if strategy is the future, policy may be the planned route to that future.

To complicate the understanding of policy still further, there can be no prederived level of where strategy and policy (if there are real differences) begin and end within organisations and their processes. It is certainly not dependent on levels of management or tiers within organisations, as was part of traditional management theory.

The very top of an organisation may develop an organisational strategy, for example at international or governmental level. In order to make that 'future' happen, there will be action necessary at many other levels below. Some organisations may develop their own strategies in order to implement the 'grand plan', whereas others may develop implementation policies. Again, it depends on terms and their usage. There is, however, a desire to make something happen, with an explanation of how to do it. This question can be best understood as wanting to bring about some form of change in a situation. If change is desired, it implies that the *status quo* presents a problem for which change is considered desirable (or necessary). A development of this thinking starts to offer some clues to an understanding of the nature of policy/strategy and the theoretical basis underpinning policy, which can in turn offer frameworks for both developing and analysing policy.

Although the term 'problem' is used here in relation to change and policy, it should not be assumed that, in this context, problems need to possess any form of negative connotation. If anything, the concept concerns change and solutions. Put simply, policy can be about making things happen to bring about change and solutions in response to a situation that can be described in terms of a problem (Hurst, 1993). Having arrived at this basic position, it follows that theoretical approaches to problem-solving can also be used in this whole area to develop and analyse policy.

Within any organisational setting, there are both internal and external components to the reasons for developing policy. There may be policy responses by an organisation to situations or events in the external world that it wishes to do something about, change or plan action for by setting out its position; this can be described as a response to policy. Equally, an organisation may wish to bring about change externally but for its own internal reasons, which can be described as developmental policy. This situation is not as complex as it may initially appear. Any organisation, or part of it, has purposes and functions (or missions). It will develop policy or plans to enable those purposes to be fulfilled. It will also develop policy in response to the external world, again to enable it to fulfil its purposes. A problem-solving/change perspective can be used in considering the basic issues of policy.

Although the problem-solving framework is now universally familiar in nursing, it is not unique to nursing. There is a vast literature in itself on theories of problem-solving (Hunt, 1996), many approaches relating to theories in behavioural psychology. These involve environmental assessment, identifying and defining the situation for change, planning the appropriate action to bring about that change, executing that plan and measuring the effectiveness. These steps can be seen as being fundamental to development and the learning of problem-solving skills or, to put it more simply, making things happen for a reason.

WHY HAVE NURSING STRATEGY OR POLICY?

In order to address this question, there are some basic assumptions about the nature of nursing. It is also worth taking time to give some consideration to nursing not just as a word or concept, but as the thing that nurses do – nursing practice, in all of its facets and dimensions, is the product of nurses and nursing.

Again, there is a vast literature on the nature of and models of nursing. As examples, the combined models of Nightingale (1859), Henderson (1978) and Orem (1987) give clear concepts of what nursing is all about, each in their own way building upon the strengths of the other (Riehl and Roy, 1974; von der Peet, 1995). Overall, nursing makes a positive and desirable contribution to individuals, humanity and health as a result of applying its specific and unique body of knowledge to individuals and situations. Nursing makes people better across a range of scenarios, health care settings in particular.

Globally, the demand for health (and thus health care) is infinite, while the resource for and supply of health is finite. At a humanitarian but also society-efficient level, effective nursing is optimising nursing for health gain. A nursing strategy is something descriptive in terms of what that contribution is – or could be – by creating an optimal vision of nursing in a future setting, retaining the knowledge and skill of nursing to make the world a better place (DoH, 1989).

In this context, policy can become the response and planned action for realising those goals. The external and internal policy elements previously discussed become policy, external in terms of what nursing should be doing and internal in terms of what nursing is and will do. Policy will be developed as a response to what is happening in the external world/environment. Policy will also be developed internally as a result of purpose and mission, and between these two positions, there will always be an overlap and a continuum. Put more simply, policy will result from the impact of the outside world on the organisation and the impact of that organisation on the world.

INTERNATIONAL PERSPECTIVES OF THE ENVIRONMENT WITHIN WHICH NURSES WORK

Nursing often slips into the protectionism/defensive mode rather than taking the pragmatic perspective that nurses have something to contribute to the health of people and discussing how that can be optimised. A very brief review of the international perspective of the nursing world shows both common threads and wide differences.

In the World Health Organisation's Targets for Health for All (WHO, 1985), the quotation of Halfdan Mahler, then Director-General, concerning the difference that nurses can make around the world is frequently quoted. Another not so frequently cited quotation made by Dr Mahler (WHO, 1985) at this time is:

> The world does indeed need nurses... it needs nurses who can diagnose community health problems and institute measures to protect, advance and monitor the health of populations as a whole, nurses who can care for the sick or disabled, nurses who can teach people to care for themselves.

From the range of skills, knowledge and competences that were highlighted here, over 20 years ago, it is clear that this concept of the 'nurse' was also about educated professional nursing.

Quite apart from the sociological definitions of a profession (Carr-Saunders and Wilson, 1933) viewed from the international perspective, the development of professional nursing means different things in different places around the world – and that is how it should be. This is because nurses adapt to meet the specific health needs and cultural environment of the population of their own countries. A challenge for the health services is how to maximise the contribution that nurses can make to health gain and unit care.

INTERNATIONAL TRENDS

For some nurses in the Western world, the development of nursing is quite advanced, with initial nursing education at baccalaureate level and accessible continuing education up to and beyond doctoral level advancing practice. There is much diversity. In Europe, there are agreed competences for the basic level generalist nurses, yet in some of the newly independent European states, nursing knowledge and formalised basic nursing education are in their infancy. It should not be assumed that the standards of practice, education and regulation are universal. There are still countries in Europe with no formal regulation, and standard-setting has only recently begun to develop standard frameworks for basic nursing education. This is being addressed through the WHO Europe's Nursing Education Strategy (WHO, 1998b).

With changing political scenarios, nursing frequently has to adapt and overcome new challenges. Nurses in some of the Western Pacific region have developed extensive clinical management roles in advanced nursing practice where scarce resources and geography necessitate their providing a full range of primary health care services. Yet in parts of South East Asia, working largely in hospital, as many nurses do, in terms of providing mainly curative and rehabilitative care to individuals, nursing practice is not always allowed to realise its full potential, despite diploma level training after 10 years of general education.

The television programme *ER* (Emergency Room) is not a realistic example of nursing's professional development and advanced nursing practice in North America. In reality, nursing has developed within the overall philosophies of health care in the USA and Canada. Nurses in the USA, through the American Nurses Association, backed the health reforms of the former Clinton administration, which, while these were not implemented because of opposition pressure, positioned nursing in relation to corporate America. The formal backing of President Clinton again reinforced the position of nurses within the overall climate of US politics. It is easy then to see the varying place of nurses and nursing within and across the political divides.

There is discussion within nursing internationally on the roles of and boundaries between nursing, medicine and other professions exploring issues of collaborative practice (ICN, 1997). The current development of HMOs is creating tension that will be interesting to observe externally. For example, in North America, some of the nursing issues also relate to the relationship or balance of power between the doctor (or 'physician' to use the North American term) and the nurse.

Nurses expand and extend their role whenever there is a shortage of medical personnel, and doctors seek to take back territory when they show a surplus. With the development of family practitioners, the power of community nurses is diminishing (Hennessy, 1997).

In the UK in 1998, the potential for nurses to lead primary health care groups as part of health reform was another contrasting development. Health reform in Canada has mirrored that of many countries, with nursing structures disappearing, multiskilling and workforce re-engineering and fiscally driven reform.

Professional nursing has its own meaning in some countries in the African region, where conflict and war situations clearly have wide-ranging implications for how and what nursing and nurses do.

This quick look around the world at what is essentially the nature and state of nursing has only scratched at the surface. It sets the context of nursing, its policy, the international context and how nursing is going to face and address the health challenges of the future.

THE HEALTH CHALLENGES

Some of the other contemporary health challenges relate to:

- global change
- demographic changes
- epidemiological changes
- new and emerging diseases
- advances in science and medical technology
- infinite demand and finite resources.

These challenges are diverse, ranging from the high-tech complexities of transplant surgery to basic infection control or, in some areas, even organising the digging of latrines to improve sanitation and public health. In the broadest sense, nursing policy in the international context must be about setting the content and context of nursing to address health issues at that level. Let us first consider some of the global health issues.

The 1995 WHO World Health Report (WHO, 1995a) saw the elimination of poverty and social deprivation as being central to health potential, as well as social and economic productivity. By 1996 the WHO World Health Report (WHO, 1996b), saw issues such as the increasing elderly population, new and emerging disease, infectious diseases and resistant organisms, and issues of child and maternal health as the global health challenges. These demanded an altered approach to health care and a response from health professionals. In 1997, the emphasis had shifted towards chronic conditions as a result of the lengthening of life expectancy and changes in lifestyle.

More recently, the 1998 World Health Report (WHO, 1998a) presented a vision for health in the 21st century, citing the reduction of the premature death rate as being one of the greatest health challenges facing humanity at the beginning of the 21st century. Although global life expectancy is reaching new heights, 21 million people face premature death during the current year (2 out of every 5 world wide, of whom 10 million will be children who will not reach their fifth birthday; WHO, 1998a).

From a review of the past 50 years of WHO data and projections of future health trends, the present priorities (Brundtland, 1998) are seen as being to:

- Roll back and where possible eradicate communicable disease, and particularly malaria from which 3,000 children are dying daily in parts of the African sub-continent.
- Fight and reduce the burden of non-communicable disease, citing tobacco-related diseases specifically.
- Help countries build sustainable health systems that can help reach equity targets and render quality services to all, with particular emphasis on the situation of women and mothers.

Nursing should have a major contribution to make in the areas of communicable diseases and infection control, health promotion and child and maternal health.

Although each WHO report had a distinct and different clinical/client group emphasis, the common thread was the need for changed approaches to health care and a response from health professionals in inter-, intra- and multidisciplinary terms to address the challenges to global health.

Global health status is not the only challenge facing nursing. Scanning the environment in which nursing currently exists, other issues also emerge:

- radical change brought about by economic constraints and health care reforms
- nurses everywhere having to change practice so that more can be achieved with decreasing resources

- differences within the global community in terms of degree and cultural appropriateness in approaches to issues including health care
- the continued emphasis on cost-effective approaches to health care demanding evidence of the value of care in order to stay in the market.

From the major challenges identified, there are opportunities for nursing and a clear role for nurses to fill on the global health agenda.

WHO GLOBAL ADVISORY GROUP

Following the World Health Assembly in 1992, the WHO Global Advisory Group on nursing and midwifery was established to advise the Director-General on all nursing and midwifery services, particularly on:

- developing mechanisms for assessing national nursing and midwifery service needs
- assisting countries with the development of national action plans for nursing and midwifery services, including research and resource planning
- monitoring progress in strengthening nursing and midwifery in support of strategies for health for all.

The Group's work resulted in the resolution carried at the 1996 World Health Assembly to strengthen nursing and midwifery (WHO, 1996a).

Some of the key elements to be strengthened related to the involvement of nurses in health reform and policy development at the national state level, nursing and midwifery education, particularly concerning primary care, and in relation to the range of human resource issues. What emerges through the more recently identified priorities is that nursing action to meet global health challenges can be viewed not just in terms of organisations but also of direct care and individual clinical practice.

ANALYSING REALITY

As a simple tool of analysis, the technique known as SWOT analysis can be applied to current situation nursing options for action in terms of Strengths, Weaknesses, Opportunities and Threats (Figure 4.1).

Strengths	**Weaknesses**
● the unique nature of nursing and its knowledge base	● how nurses demonstrate the value of nursing ● the secondary care domination of health care systems ● nursing education
Opportunities	**Threats**
● WHO Health for All Renewal (WHO, 1997) ● recognition of the potential of nursing and midwifery ● Global Advisory Group Resolution (WHO, 1996a) 1996 ● the position of nursing within health reform	● nursing not fulfilling its potential contribution ● a surplus of physicians ● a resistance to change in nursing ● the position of nursing within health reform

Figure 4.1   SWOT analysis of nursing options for action

Considering the strengths, weaknesses, opportunities and threats for nursing at the moment, and faced with the type of health challenges highlighted in the successive World Health reports, a logical conclusion must be that there is a global need for the strengthening of nursing and midwifery in order to make the most effective use of nursing for health gain. The global health challenges are well documented and described as some of the options for action. In addition, there is a clear recognition, at least in terms of formal statements if not policy, that there is a role for nursing. The question remains, however, whether or not nursing is seen in the process of developing solutions to some of these health challenges or problems.

Work undertaken by the WHO Expert Committee on Nursing Practice (WHO, 1995b) was quite clear in its recommendation in terms of not addressing the issues of nursing practice at the global/international level as approaches to issues should be country specific, and, more importantly, that nursing was squarely placed in terms of 'available human resources for health and the division of labour among all health care personnel'. The emphasis was placed upon a policy for the development of nursing as 'an integral part of human resource development'. This complements the contemporary management thinking, which ensures that strategic human resource development is positioned in relation to core business objectives.

One of the interesting things in the international arena is the use of language – its meaning and understanding – and use of words. The health business, particularly through the process of health reform, has built up its own code of language and management terms. This is reflected in the discussion in these paragraphs.

The world has moved on significantly since the original Alma Ata Declaration in 1978 (WHO, 1978) and the Health for All by the Year 2000 (WHO, 1979). Now the language is about Health for All Renewal and Health for All in the 21st century. What is clear is that the overall, and longer-term, assessment of global health needs and problem identification will form part of Health for All Renewal (Bankjowski *et al.*, 1997).

INTERNATIONAL NURSING POLICY PERSPECTIVES

There is no simple answer to the basic question of what is meant by international nursing policy. Describing historical events relevant to the subject does not present the full picture. Mintzberg (1994), in considering strategy development, describes the way in which the obvious evolves and does not clearly differentiate between policy and strategy (see the discussion of the difference between policy and strategy above). Taking the issue of professionalism and professions controlling their own destiny, it might be that nursing policy will emerge naturally as the obvious path to be taken to achieve identifiable goals and solve health problems. It may not matter whether nursing policy is always formalised at a particular level; the important issue is the ability of nursing and nurses to influence the development of solutions. Without a policy framework, however, including values and goals, the contextual framework for that influence may be lacking.

The policy analysis framework of problem-solving quoted earlier uses problem-solving with the following elements:

- problem identification
- problem assessment
- planning interventions
- implementation
- evaluation.

These elements also form a framework for policy development and analysis. Nursing practice (the product) is supported and enabled through organisation and education. In terms of achieving effective outcomes it was exactly this policy model that was applied by Nightingale in that safe (and effective) nursing was the product of the organisation of nurses and the application of knowledge through education.

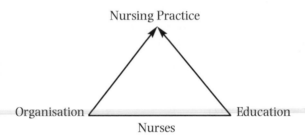

Figure 4.2   Nursing policy model

With significant amounts of work and policy development being undertaken in these areas by a number of agencies, international nursing policy develops within a coherent framework capable of analysis and with the ownership of the profession. It is this free policy development that can be interpreted and translated through nursing structures in all settings that illustrates the process of international nursing policy. Furthermore, nurses are seeking no longer to operate in isolation but to understand the need to develop in the context of multiple settings and agencies.

Nursing is well down the line in developing policy to address some of the major health issues that have been identified by the WHO (see above). This clearly relates to the role of nursing practice in addressing the global health challenges. The role of nursing can be clearly specified and articulated in this respect.

AND SO TO THE FUTURE

Some of the challenges facing nursing are also opportunities, and nursing needs to look at how it can accommodate and assimilate such change. Fortunately, for many nurses, their role concerns learning new skills, adjusting their thinking and practice, and realising that high levels of uncertainty and change are the norm.

Nursing and its policy development needs to think and work more in the multidisciplinary context and also in terms of interdisciplinary partnerships. This does not detract from the uniqueness of nursing. In fact, it is enhanced when nurses share their skill and accumulated knowledge and evidence with other members of the health care team. Rather than being territorial over what is or is not the role of nurses, some acknowledgement needs to be given to what nurses are doing in many parts of the world. There are nurses determining their own scope of nursing practice, who is the most appropriate person to be the care-giver and what is the appropriate educational preparation for that practice. This could be regarded as nursing policy: applying knowledge, making human resource decisions in care management and continuing adjustment of the educational provision.

When nursing policy is successful, as for example in some of the primary health care settings in developing countries, this is because even where functional overlap exists, it does not present a threat or 'competition' for other health care workers. It is about meeting health needs within resources available – not just in terms of money, but also in terms of people, ability and knowledge. Flexibility, competence and confidence are also keys to the future. These will be enhanced by shared learning or health professionals learning together, understanding each other, and by sharing skills.

Set also in the context of the post-capitalist world, the democracy and answerability that society now demands of political structures will be translated into work patterns, and in nursing it will increasingly concern accountability. Accountability is not just about professional practice and conduct, but also about giving value for money and accepting personal responsibility.

It will be through this type of framework and embracing these environmental factors that international nursing policy will continue to develop and evolve further. It may not be the policy of any one formal body or institution but a framework and amalgam of policy – solutions offered by nursing to meet the challenges to health. Nursing policy will be part of political structures and systems – the challenge being for nursing to make its optimum contribution globally to the health and well-being of the world's people.

REFERENCES

Bankjowski, Z., Bryant, J.H. and Gallagher, J. (1997) Ethics, Equity and the Renewal of WHO's Health for All Strategy: Proceedings of the 29th CIOMS

Conference. Geneva: Council for International Organizations of Medical Science (CIOMS).

Brundtland, G.H. (1998) *Speech to Fifty-first World Health Assembly*, Geneva, 13 May, 1998. (A51/DIV/6). Geneva: WHO.

Carr-Saunders, A.N. and Wilson, P.A. (1933) *The Professions*. Oxford: Clarendon Press.

Department of Health (1989) *A Strategy for Nursing*. London: HMSO.

Henderson, V. (1978) *Basic Principles of Nursing*. New York: Macmillan.

Hennessy, D. (1997) Proceedings of International Nursing Policy Seminar, University of Birmingham, (unpublished).

Hunt, J. (1996) *Nursing Policy into Action* paper presented at RCN Annual Conference, October, 1996 (unpublished).

Hurst, K. (1993) *Problem-solving in Nursing Practice*. London: Scutari Press.

International Council of Nurses (1997) *Proceedings of Council of National Representatives Meeting*, Vancouver, Canada. Geneva: ICN.

Mintzberg, H. (1994) *The Rise and Fall of Strategic Planning*. New York: Prentice Hall.

Mintzberg, H. and Quinn, J.B. (1991) *The Strategy Process: Concepts, Context and Cases*, 2nd edn. Engelwood Cliffs, NJ: Prentice Hall.

Nightingale, F. (1859) *Notes on Nursing*. London: Longman.

Orem, D. (1987) *Nursing: Concepts of Practice*. New York: McGraw Hill.

Riehl, J.P. and Roy, C. (1974) *Conceptual Models for Nursing Practice*. New York: Appleton Century Crofts.

von der Peet, R. (1995) *The Nightingale Model of Nursing*. Edinburgh: Campion.

WHO (1978) *Alma Ata 1978: Primary Health Care*. Geneva: WHO.

WHO (1979) *Formulating Strategies for Health for All by the Year 2000*. Geneva: WHO.

WHO (1985) *Targets for Health for All*. Copenhagen: WHO.

WHO (1995a) *World Health Report*. Geneva: WHO.

WHO (1995b) *Nursing Practice: Report of the WHO Expert Committee*. Geneva: WHO.

WHO (1996a) *Forty-ninth World Health Assembly* Agenda item 17, Strengthening nursing and midwifery. Geneva: WHO.

WHO (1996b) *The World Health Report* 1998. Geneva: WHO.

WHO (1997) *The World Health Report* 1998. Geneva: WHO.

WHO (1998a) *The World Health Report* 1998. Geneva: WHO.

WHO Europe (1998b) *WHO European Office Nursing Education Strategy*. Copenhagen: WHO EURO.

Public health at European level – a new challenge for nurses?

A historical approach

Christopher Birt

Editors' Introduction

This chapter provides an important description of nursing in the EU, tracing its history from nursing in Roman Catholic institutions to the establishment of the Permanent Committee of Nurses in 1971, with formal recognition from the European Commission for it to be its advisory committee on nursing. Nevertheless, the Commission did not identify a useful role for nurses or nursing organisations in public health. This is an interesting case study illustrating how effective lobbying in the late 1960s included a nursing voice as a formal advisory committee to the EU. Twenty years later, however, the Commission does not appear to have sought a nursing voice for public health in the EU, nor is it clear whether nurses have lobbied sufficiently to be included. There is a challenge here for nurses to grasp the opportunities offered.

INTRODUCTION

In 1992, it was estimated that there were 1,700,000 registered nurses in the EU, which at that time still consisted only of 12 member states as Austria, Sweden and Finland had not yet joined. However, the nurse-to-citizen ratio varied considerably in 1991 in smaller member states, ranging from 25,000 nurses for a population of 10,000,000 in Portugal to 28,000 nurses for 3,500,000 people in Ireland, and 4,000 nurses for the population of 378,000 in Luxembourg. In larger member states, 295,000 nurses were serving 56,000,000 French people, while 470,000 nurses were working for 79,000,000 Germans, and in the UK there were 590,000 nurses for a population of 57,000,000. Although substantially a female profession throughout the EU, the percentage of female nurses in 1991 varied from 97 per cent in Denmark, 83 per cent in Portugal and 82 per cent in Germany, to 75 per cent in Luxembourg. The extent of part-time working also varied widely, being 1.5 per cent in Ireland, 5 per cent in Spain, 48 per cent in the Netherlands and 69 per cent in Portugal (Hospital Committee of the European Community, 1992; Evers, 1996).

Although nursing today constitutes a major professional group throughout the EU, the origins and traditions of the profession vary markedly between member states. Convergence has been rapid in recent years, and this trend is set to continue now that there is a common pattern of training throughout the EU, with (at least theoretically) free movement for employment purposes for all trained nurses throughout all member states (Quinn and Russell, 1993).

HISTORY OF NURSING IN WESTERN EUROPE

In the Middle Ages, the provision of care was very much associated with the Roman Catholic monastic institutions and with the infirmaries that were attached to some monasteries. Hence, caring was seen as one of the expected roles of monks and, even more so, of nuns (Godfrey, 1955; Dainton, 1961). In some EU member states with an uninterrupted Roman Catholic tradition, this tradition has been carried on into the 20th century, and nuns continue to work as nurses in some hospitals.

However, in much of northern Europe, the monasteries, and the infirmaries associated with them, were closed as a result of the Reformation, mainly in the 16th and 17th centuries (Dainton, 1961). Meanwhile, starting somewhat before the beginning of the Industrial Revolution, there began to be a general renaissance of interest across northern Europe in various aspects of medical practice, and between 1700 and 1900 large hospitals were built in most large towns and cities. The staffing of these institutions at first often did not include nurses but was limited to physicians, surgeons and apothecaries, who usually visited on a daily basis. However, carers were subsequently recruited to carry out nursing functions, albeit with full accountability to the medical staff. These 'nurses' lacked not only training, but also any form of professional ethos or background to their work, and they were not generally held in high repute at that time. There are many accounts of drunkenness and orgies involving these caring staff of the hospitals, and it was indeed normal for wages to be paid at least partly in the form of beer. For example, at St Thomas' Hospital in London in 1838, nurses received nine shillings and sevenpence (approximately 48p, or ECU 0.6 in today's money) each week, in addition to a free supply of beer, as wages (Abel-Smith, 1964; St Thomas' Hospital, 1969).

This was the world of nursing that Florence Nightingale observed and which she set out to reform. Her drive and initiative can be identified as the principal origins of nursing as we now understand it – an indispensable component of the health services provided by a professional group held almost universally in high esteem (Abel-Smith, 1964). However, others also contributed significantly to these reforms. In Germany, it was a Protestant minister, Pastor Fliedner, and his wife who re-established nursing as a profession. To give young women entering this profession a better status than that enjoyed by other hospital carers, he gave them the ecclesiastical status of 'deaconess' – almost a throw-back to the care by nuns in the pre-Reformation infirmaries. However, Fliedner's nursing service was taken over by the Red Cross and experienced a major setback, partly on account of medical domination (Weinrich, 1993).

One of the most significant features of the Nightingale reforms was the establishment of an independent profession free from medical domination (Abel-Smith, 1964). Most of the main features of these reforms were rapidly adopted by the countries of western Europe, including both the German and Austro-Hungarian empires. It is of passing interest to note that they were never espoused within the Russian empire. It is probably as a consequence of this that nurses always had low status in the successor Union of Socialist Soviet Republics and that they usually still today remain the handmaidens of doctors in all member states of the Commonwealth of Independent States (Birt *et al.*, 1999).

In 1899, Ethel Bedford Fenwick established the ICN. Forty-six years later, as the Second World War drew to a close, many European nurses began to express a wish for a European professional identity and, in 1946, in London, a meeting of the presidents of 28 national associations of nurses was held. Internationalism within nursing became the order of the day and, in 1953, the UK's Royal College of Nursing joined the Northern Nurses Federation, the other members of which included Belgium, France, the Netherlands, Switzerland and Luxembourg. This grouping subsequently renamed itself the Western European Nursing Group (Quinn, 1993).

   In 1957, the original Treaty of Rome was signed, which set up the
original European Economic Community (EEC), and the intention that
there should be a free movement of professionals such as nurses within
all member states became evident. The president of the ICN at that
time, Alice Clamargeran, made contact with the newly established
European Commission, which was starting to prepare draft directives
for professional groups, including nurses. This led to a lengthy but
constructive dialogue with Commission officials, led on behalf of the
nurses by Nelly Goffard, president of the Belgian Nurses Federation.
These relationships and discussions were maintained until the
Standing Committee of Nurses (which is known, confusingly, as the
PCN – Permanent Committee of Nurses) was established in 1971 with
formal recognition from the Commission for its being its advisory
committee on nursing (Quinn, 1993).

NURSING DIRECTIVES

The first draft texts of these Directives were submitted for comment to
the European Parliament (hereafter referred to as Parliament) in 1969
and to the Economic and Social Committee in 1970. This was of
course shortly before the UK, Denmark and Ireland joined the EEC, and
nursing organisations in these countries were becoming anxious to be
involved in the discussion of the texts. Work was also proceeding on
Directives relating to other professions, and in October 1973, under
the chairmanship of Commissioner Professor Ralph Dahrendorf, a
hearing took place on the recognition of medical qualifications. Subsequent drafts of the Nursing Directives gave more attention than previously to the quality (rather than quantity) of training, and a nurse
training syllabus was attached as an appendix to the relevant draft
Directive. However, the revised text submitted to Parliament still
referred to only 3,700 hours of total training rather than the 4,600
hours favoured by the PCN, which then began intensive lobbying of
the Commission. An eventual outcome much more to the liking of the
PCN can be seen as its first major victory. The Directives were finally
agreed in 1977, and implemented 2 years later. Presumably, on
account of the assistance that had been provided by the PCN, the
Council of Ministers decided at the same time that a new Advisory
Committee on Training in Nursing should be established 'within the
Commission', which gave it automatic formal status. The Committee
has three expert members from each member state, one each from the
practising profession, from nurse training establishments and the

competent authority in the member state concerned (Standing Committee of Nurses of the EC, 1992; Quinn, 1993).

This Advisory Committee on Training in Nursing has remained highly active ever since it was set up. For example, it has reported to the Commission on the training needs of specialist nurses in a number of areas of work, including psychiatry, paediatrics, cancer care and primary health care. It has also reviewed the basic training needs of nurses responsible for general care, later adding a section to this to include primary health care within this basic training. Meanwhile, the PCN has also been active in a number of areas, including carrying out a major survey of the health services in member states and of nursing structures within these services. The PCN has also sought to maintain relationships with other relevant European organisations, most obviously including the WHO's European Office in Copenhagen (Quinn, 1993).

THE MAASTRICHT TREATY

Health ministers in European Community (EC) member states had met formally as a Health Council since the 1970s, even though the EC institutions at that time had no responsibilities in any treaty for any aspect of health or health services. In the 1980s, they agreed to collaborate (outside any treaty obligations) on a number of EC-wide public health initiatives, of which the best known are probably 'Europe Against Cancer' and 'Europe Against AIDS'. They also included lesser-known projects such as that setting out to encourage the concept of health-promoting schools in all member states. There were a total of about 15 such programmes agreed, and the Commission was asked to service these, so a Public Health Unit was set up to do this within Directorate General Five (DG V). It was therefore not surprising that, at the next Inter-governmental Conference, it was suggested and agreed that such work to promote improved public health across the future EU should at this stage be included formally within the new Treaty that was to be agreed (Birt, 1995).

This was, of course, the Maastricht Treaty, which was implemented on 1 November 1993 but which had been much discussed for at least 2 years before this. It presented a new situation to all organisations concerned with health and health care in the EU, on account of Article 129 of the amended Treaty of Rome, which, for the first time, gave the EU institutions a formal competency in the field of public health. It was inevitable, right and proper that nursing organisations should have expected to become involved in the working of these new arrangements. They were supposed to be supportive to the actions of member states and were not supposed to affect patient services themselves, but they excluded the possibility of the establishment of minimal standards in public health matters (Allman, 1993; Birt, 1995).

The Commission, which appeared to address its new responsibilities in this field somewhat tentatively and with caution, has not thus far shown much evidence of any comprehension that there is a useful role for nurses and nursing organisations in support of public health programmes. This may be, at least in part, on account of the lack of experience of practical public health within DG V itself – the Directorate General within which the new post-Maastricht Directorate of Public Health and Safety is situated. The staffing of the Directorate is very largely career civil servants (as is the case in the rest of the Commission), and there are few people within it with relevant health professional experience of their own.

Within less than a month of the implementation of the Maastricht Treaty (formally the Treaty of European Political and Monetary Union), the Commission published a discussion paper on public health (European Commission, 1993). The Commission went out of its way to explain that this should not have been seen as a strategy document – and it was indeed nothing of the kind. The paper outlined the progress made in recent years in various member states to improve public health and went on to outline the Commission's immediate intentions in this field. There were three particularly significant series of paragraphs. The first of these outlined the criteria to be applied by the Commission when it sought to prioritise possible candidate subject areas that might attract future public health funding from the EU. These criteria categorise diseases that might be candidates for EU funded programmes as follows:

- diseases that cause, in the absence of any intervention, significant premature death (years of life lost) and/or are associated with high overall death rates
- diseases that cause, or are likely to cause in the absence of intervention, significant levels of ill-health on account of an associated high prevalence of morbidity and/or serious disability (years of disability-free life lost)
- diseases that have significant implications for the quality of life in addition to major socioeconomic effects, such as high health care and treatment costs, or which are associated with considerable absenteeism and unfitness for work

- diseases for which practicable preventive measures exist
- diseases for which there would be added value from EU-funded actions, in particular on account of economies of scale.

The second significant series of statements concerned consultation mechanisms, emphasising the importance of these and the necessity of establishing appropriate new consultation mechanisms for public health in the EU in the light of its new responsibilities in this field. The paper promised that firm proposals for these mechanisms would follow, but these are currently still awaited. It is interesting to note that earlier drafts of this discussion document set out some clear ideas regarding possible consultation mechanisms, but these were omitted, for one reason or another, from the final published version.

Finally, at the end of its paper, the Commission identified eight areas in which it intended to make firm policy proposals for funded initiatives over the next 2–3 years. Some of these were a continuation into the future (and in some cases an extension) of some of the larger programmes previously agreed by member states on the basis of voluntary collaboration, but others broke new ground. The eight areas were:

- health data and information (translated from 'Eurospeak', this really means the establishment and administration of an EU public health common data set)
- health promotion
- cancer
- AIDS and other communicable diseases
- drug dependency
- intentional and unintentional accidents and injuries
- pollution-related diseases
- rare diseases.

Since the publication of this paper, the Commission has published detailed proposals in some of these areas. Commission proposals for new funded policies for cancer (European Commission, 1994a), AIDS and communicable diseases (European Commission, 1994b), drug dependency (European Commission, 1994c) and health promotion (European Commission, 1994d) have all been approved by Parliament and by the Council, and these are now operating. Those working in relevant fields anywhere in the EU may now apply for funding support provided that their initiatives comply with the requirements of each specific policy and providing that colleagues in more than one member state are collaborating on a project for which support is sought. This appears to be the Commission's practical application of the 'added value' criterion (see above). It appears, of all the stated criteria, that this is the only one that must apply in all cases.

The Commission has also published its proposals for health data and information (European Commission, 1995), in which it explains how it wishes to set up its public health data set. These have been approved by Parliament and the Council and, at the time of writing, await implementation. Commission proposals for accidents and injuries, for pollution-related diseases and for rare diseases have all been published during 1997 by the Public Health and Safety Directorate in DG V, which is situated in Luxembourg (and which is the successor to the pre-Maastricht Public Health Unit). These proposals are subject to current discussions in the Parliament and the Council.

ARE NURSES READY AND EQUIPPED TO WORK IN THE POST-MAASTRICHT EU?

As already explained, while nursing in most EU member states shares some common origins, and while there is a quite rapid convergence of nurse training and some aspects of practice, there are also considerable differences remaining concerning both the numbers of nurses per head of population and also what they do.

The conceptualisation of what health services can and should address, and which of these should be identified as developmental priorities, has taken a quantum leap since the WHO Alma Ata Conference at the end of the 1970s. This conference laid much of the basis for the development of both modern primary health care (including general practice) and modern health promotion practice (WHO, 1978). However, throughout the EU, nurse training institutions appear to have been slow to pay much more than lip-service to these new ideas and to their practical expression, and in reality in all EU member state nurses are still employed mainly in hospitals. A rapid review of the situation regarding primary health care, public health and health promotion nursing in all member states (carried out immediately before Sweden, Finland and Austria became EU members) revealed the following situation (Quinn and Russell, 1993; WHO, 1994).

Belgium

Nurses in training can choose courses in public health and public services, health education and epidemiology, or nutrition and dietetics.

However, within the health services themselves, there are as yet neither any higher nursing qualifications in these areas nor any possibility for specialisation in these areas of nursing practice. Indeed, there appear to be few opportunities in Belgium for nurses to be employed outside hospitals or nursing homes.

Denmark

Nurse training was reorganised in 1989/90, and all basic training includes the functions of the nurse in the promotion of health, the prevention of illness and rehabilitation. Postgraduate nursing diplomas are available in both public health nursing and nursing and management in the primary health care service. About one-third of nurses are employed in the community nursing care sector, most providing support to primary health care, including a 24-hour home nursing service, and public heath nurses are employed by all municipalities; they give special emphasis in their work to the needs of children.

France

In 1978, a new nursing law was passed. This included the recognition of the nurse's own specific role and her role as an auxiliary to a doctor, but it also referred to nurses' participation in prevention of illness, education, health and training. There is, however, perceived to be a considerable shortage of nurses in France and, in addition, the profession does not appear to enjoy a particularly high status in terms of public perception. In practice, there appear to be few opportunities for nurses to work in either primary health care or public health.

Germany

Basic nurse training is essentially theoretical but includes an emphasis on psychology and sociology, and a full-time 2-year postbasic course is provided in public hygiene. Nursing practice appears to have changed quite rapidly in recent years, and an increasing number of nurses now want to work outside hospitals, preferring to take more responsibility for the patients they care for in their home surroundings. Accordingly, nurses are becoming more involved in most aspects of primary health care, but not so much in public health, although the Länder (the provinces) carry formal responsibility for health education and public health in their areas.

Greece

Nurse training is based in technical education institutes, which provide a theoretically based course closely integrated with clinical teaching. For specialty training, there are seven graduate courses, usually lasting 1 year, one of which is in public health nursing. Since 1983, primary health care and public health nurses have been employed to work in health centres, which nowadays usually enjoy spacious premises. However, primary health care concepts are developing only slowly, and doctors and nurses are learning together how to promote health and how to mobilise the population to participate in its own health care.

Ireland

Nurse training is the responsibility of the Nursing Board, which recognises 32 training schools, 18 of which are for general nurse training, which includes some primary health care experience. There are also a few postbasic courses, including a 1 year course in public health nursing. Community nursing services and health visiting are, however, somewhat rudimentary throughout the country.

Italy

Basic nurse education takes place in authorised nurse training schools, and this complies with the relevant EC Directive of 1979. A number of postbasic specialist courses are also available, but other than one for health visitor training, these do not provide relevant training for community or public health nurses. Community nursing appears at present to be poorly developed, but the nursing service is currently being reorganised in line with a recent Act of Parliament (which was in fact requested by the profession itself). It is to be hoped that the potential for nurses to become more involved than in the past in public health activities may now be realised.

Luxembourg

There are four schools of nursing recognised by the Luxembourg government, and training fulfils the requirements of the Directives. Experience of home nursing is included in these courses, but there is no specialist postbasic education in any aspect of community or public health nursing. These aspects of the nursing role do not appear to be well developed, but the role of the nurse, as defined by The Grand Ducal Regulation (1983, p. 89) 'includes participation in education, training, management, health promotion and prevention, hygiene and the development and application of measures to control infection and contagion'. The nurse's role also includes activities that contribute to the 'protection and maintenance of health or recovery from illness and restoration of vital functions, and to health promotion'.

The Netherlands

Basic nurse training is well developed in the Netherlands and includes routine experience in general hospitals, psychiatric hospitals, nursing homes, institutions for the mentally handicapped and areas of community care. Postbasic education in both community nursing and community psychiatric nursing is available. Nurses work in a wide variety of health care settings, some as independent practitioners. Community nursing is well developed, and in 1986 the number of inhabitants per community nurse was calculated to be 2,910.

Portugal

Nurse training prepares students to provide nursing care at three levels – those of the individual, the family and the community – and includes exposure to management of the health services. Before entering post-basic education, students must have completed 2 years of professional experience since qualification. There are postbasic courses in eight specialties, two being public health nursing and rehabilitation nursing. Community nursing is well developed, and nurses are usually included on the management boards of health centres. They also play a part in all aspects of primary health care.

Spain

Since nurse training became a university-based activity (the first university course being instigated in 1980), nurse education has become much more closely related to the health needs of the population than had previously been the case, featuring within the curriculum public health features together with statistics, demography and epidemiology. Postbasic specialist nurse education is available for seven specialties, including community health care nursing. Nursing within primary health care is well developed in Spain, and nurses, usually operating within primary health care teams, provide services to individuals, families and communities, utilising programmes of health promotion, the prevention of disease, cure and rehabilitation.

United Kingdom

Nurse training has in recent years become increasingly a university-based activity. A new scheme for nurse education ('Project 2000') was introduced in 1989; this emphasises 'holistic care' that is planned to meet the physical, emotional and social needs of the whole person, whether in hospital or in the community. There is also a considerable emphasis on health promotion. After registration, there are many opportunities for both academic and clinically based further education, up to and including Master's or doctoral programmes in, for example, district nursing or health visiting. Nurses play a major role in all community health services, including being community (district) nurses, health visitors, practice nurses and midwives.

What conclusions can one draw from this rapid review of nursing training and practice across the EU? The main conclusion is that a profession that grew up mainly to provide caring services to sick patients has been trying, with differing degrees of success across the EU, to reform its educational and service practices to make nursing more relevant than hitherto to the health needs of the people. It has placed an emphasis on health promotion and rehabilitation, based in the community, in addition to caring for the sick. However, there appears to be still a long way to go, and nursing has clearly been trying to identify its appropriate role within post-Alma Ata primary health care (WHO, 1978), the context of Health for All and the 38 targets defined by the European Region of WHO with reference to Health for All (WHO, 1985). The underlying concepts behind these new primary health care and public health movements still appear not to be fully understood in depth by many within the nursing profession, including some nurse teachers.

Moreover, the opportunities offered within the EU for nurses in different member states to learn from each other are not being exploited as much as they should be. Perhaps, in addition to a further consideration of curriculum issues, as referred to above in relation to primary health care and Health for All (WHO, 1978, 1985), nurse training institutions should also give increasing attention to computer literacy, language skills and placements for students in other member states (S. McBean, personal communication, 1996).

IS NURSING RESPONDING TO THE POST-MAASTRICHT OPPORTUNITIES?

The immediate answer to this question would appear to be a negative one; there is little evidence that nurses working in the health services operating in member states, as described above, have responded in any positive way to the new EU public health policies emanating from Luxembourg or to the funding opportunities that these policies provide. Nor is there much evidence that nursing organisations within member states have played much of a part in the development of these new policies or in discussions relating to them.

However, this is certainly not for lack of leadership from the PCN, which has clearly sought to place the nursing profession at the vanguard of EU public health developments. Perhaps it has been let down by nursing colleagues working within the limits of their parochial views in the various member states. In a policy statement issued in 1992 (Standing Committee of Nurses of the EC, 1992), the PCN declared that its stated objectives are:

- to study and take action within its competence on matters relating to the nursing profession and the delivery of health care in the EU
- to present its opinions and recommendations on all matters within its competence to the EU institutions and to take any action it deems appropriate to ensure that these are duly considered
- to seek to influence the Commission and the Advisory Committees of the Council of the EU on behalf of and in the interests of the nursing profession of the EU
- to provide a database about the nursing profession within the member states and to bring such information to the attention of the EU institutions and national nursing organisations
- to be instrumental in bringing about and furthering the co-operation between international health organisations, research institutions and the EU
- to liaise with the Committees or other bodies representing other health care professions at EU level.

At the same time, the PCN also issued a fascinating statement concerning its basic philosophy and beliefs (Standing Committee of Nurses of the EC, 1994), which was to the effect that:

- health is a state of complete physical, mental and social well-being that is influenced by several aspects of society, for example the economy, housing, employment, the environment and technology

- health policy should be based on a health care system that is continuously adapting to developments in society and thus to the need of the population for the highest obtainable conditions of health promotion, treatment and care
- society should contribute to assisting the ability of the individual to participate actively in all areas of life in order to improve his own lifestyle to the optimum possible
- the contribution of nursing should rank as an essential element of national health plans, and nurses should participate in the debate on health policy
- legislation for nursing practice should recognise the nurse's contribution to the organisation, development and delivery of health care. It should be formulated to maximise the nurse's ability to meet the health needs of the population
- nursing education is a continuum that includes basic education for licensure, clinical experience, education in specialty areas and continuing and advanced education
- all basic programmes of nursing should prepare generalist nurses, who are able to function in both hospital and community. All specialist knowledge and skills subsequently acquired should be built on this foundation. Candidates for nursing education should have completed a full secondary education and have qualifications for admission equivalent to those required for higher education
- nursing research provides a knowledge and understanding of factors for the promotion of health, the prevention of illness and the improvement of nursing practice.

At the same time, the PCN (Standing Committee of Nurses of the EC, 1992) stated that it recognised that:

- health policy and health related issues would occupy an increasing part of the EU agenda
- the Single European Market would affect the delivery of health care in the member states
- nurses should exert all possible influence on the formulation of health policy in the EU.

In the final part of this statement, the PCN stated its intention to pursue its objectives in its policy areas by carrying out a number of stated activities. These included maintaining a presence in Brussels, maintaining an awareness of the Commission's activities, keeping in regular touch with appropriate contacts within relevant parts of the

Commission, providing information to the Commission and seeking EU funding for nursing-related conferences and projects (Standing Committee of the Nurses of the EC, 1992).

The PCN has in this way demonstrated the clear lead it is attempting to provide to a (possibly foot-dragging) nursing profession across the whole EU. The PCN has shown that it at least has a clear under-standing of the principles of the new public health, of Health for All and of post-Alma Ata primary health care. It also has a vision of the extent to which health care will be increasingly influenced by decisions taken at EU level, and of the increasing significance in the future of EU-led public health programmes. Finally, the PCN has identified the role that nurses can and should be playing in the development of policies and practice in these various fields. It is indeed sad and unfortunate that, so far at least, the part being played by nurses does not in reality fulfil these expectations.

Since the issuing of the various policy statements already referred to, the PCN has published some more specialist documents in which its philosophy and thinking are developed further. One such document provides a European perspective on the nurse's contribution to the care of the elderly (Standing Committee of Nurses of the EC, 1993a) in which implications for nursing care across the EU are explored in six areas: health promotion, health maintenance, acute care, rehabilitation, care of the seriously ill and dying, and the education, research and policy development activities relevant to all these aspects of nursing practice.

A second document sets out the views of the PCN on the nurse's contribution to EU public health policy (Standing Committee of Nurses of the EC, 1993b). This states clearly that a public health policy for Europe should be based on the following principles:

- It must be based on the Health for All targets, and should incorporate the declaration of Alma Ata
- It must promote a change of emphasis away from hospital treatment services to those concerned with prevention and health promotion
- It must address the need for the creation of a climate of public health in which health-promoting determinants can be introduced into policy development in areas that affect communities, homes and families, and into the context of strategies to address poverty, discrimination, poor housing and pollution
- It should emphasise the need to create healthy and health-promoting work environments

- It must address the need to decrease the consumption of tobacco, alcohol and other drugs
- It must address a number of issues relating to reproductive and sexual health
- It must tackle the special needs of vulnerable groups, including children, the elderly, the mentally ill, the mentally handicapped and the homeless.

A further publication in 1994, on *Public Health after Maastricht* (Standing Committee of Nurses of the EC, 1994), reaffirmed these principles in the context of the new possibilities for EU-led health activities. This document, recognising the fact that EU public health programmes can work successfully only if a wide range of agencies collaborate effectively in order to achieve agreed goals, stressed the importance of nursing interests (including the PCN itself) being involved in both the planning and the delivery of such programmes. It also identified (perhaps in 1994, with considerable foresight) the significant role that the European Parliament was likely to play in the establishment of EU public health programmes. It identified the need for nursing interests to play a part in informing and educating MEPs about health issues generally and to become involved in lobbying at the parliamentary level. The document also encouraged the EU institutions to start to consider the public health implications of enlarging the EU by accepting central European states as new members. It indicated that the Public Health and Safety Directorate in DG V needed to recruit more staff from the health professions themselves if it were to make coherent sense of its new public health responsibilities. The publication also suggested that each member state should provide to the Directorate, on an annual basis, a report on health needs and on progress in relation to EU public health target areas.

THE AMSTERDAM TREATY AND ITS IMPLICATIONS FOR NURSES

In 1997, the EU completed its next great leap forward. Such strides are achieved at Inter-governmental Conferences, which are held every few years to review progress towards (in the words of the Treaty of Rome) 'ever closer union' and chart developments over the subsequent few years. Maastricht had provided the climax for the previous Inter-governmental Conference: this had brought public health into the EU. The next one was completed at Amsterdam in June 1997 (Treaty on

European Union, 1997). Not long before the Conference began, there was still no general expectation that the new (Maastricht) public health powers would be altered so soon after their adoption – but then came the bovine spongiform encephalopathy crisis. The Parliament adopted a report that was strongly critical both of the EC and the UK government of the day. Indeed, the Parliament even threatened to sack the whole Commission. This brought its President, Jacques Santer, to address Parliament in contrite mood when he stated that, in future, 'health must be at the forefront of the development of Europe' (European Commission, 1997). Since then, the EC has been reviewing how to improve its own management of public health hazards and programmes designed to respond to these. At the same time, it proposed substantially increased public health powers for the Intergovernmental Conference. These initial proposals were watered down considerably, but the Amsterdam Treaty text (now subject to ratification) includes, among other changes, the possibility for the EU institutions in future to legislate to harmonise, in certain limited fields, laws relating to public health protection across all member states.

If more power and responsibility in the public health field is soon to be exerted at EU level, it becomes even more important for nurses to begin to play their full and rightful part in the Brussels and Luxembourg decision-making scene. There is plenty of scope for this. The European public health organisations, the European Public Health Alliance (EPHA), the Association of Schools of Public Health in the European Region (ASPHER) and the European Public Health Association (EUPHA) are becoming much more influential; a suitable starting point would be for nurses to become fully involved in these organisations. Those working in academic departments of nursing with close relationships with medical schools could take a lead in ensuring that their universities played a full part in ASPHER. Nurses involved in teaching or research should all join EUPHA (in the UK by joining the Society for Social Medicine), for which they will receive their own copies of the *European Journal of Public Health*. Attendance at EUPHA meetings can lead to real involvement in policy-making activities. Similarly, nurses can seek to encourage any non-governmental organisations in which they are involved (which could be health authorities, Trusts or community health councils) to join EPHA, or they can join themselves as individual members. EUPHA, ASPHER and EPHA are together constructing a 'European Public Health Platform', within which there should be a nursing presence. The platform seems likely to become a significant player in future policy development.

CONCLUSION

The nursing profession in Europe has worked hard over the past quarter of a century to modernise its training programmes and to work closely and effectively with the EC to bring a degree of uniformity and order to nurse training and practice throughout the EU. The nursing organisations in member states had the foresight to set up an effective PCN that has achieved a great deal for the profession. It continues to show an ability to offer leadership to rest of the profession (Williams, 1996a), as for example demonstrated by the radical ideas that emerged from the recent Inter-governmental Conference (RCN, 1996; Williams, 1996b), which culminated in the Amsterdam Treaty (Treaty on European Union, 1997).

But has the PCN moved ahead too fast for most nursing colleagues in member states? There appears to be reason to question the extent to which the underlying concepts of Health for All, and therefore of policy development springing from Health for All, are really understood and accepted by most nurses. There is certainly scant evidence that nurses are playing the part they could play in the new public health, either in member states or at EU level. Even where public health nursing is well developed, this appears to be in most cases concerned with programmes aimed at individuals. There is little evidence that nurses have grasped opportunities to involve themselves in population programmes, or that they are addressing health protection issues in any serious or coherent manner. As already stated, they should now seek to address the challenges of the post-Amsterdam situation.

At EU level, the PCN has identified a clear path for constructive nursing involvement in the new and developing public health programmes, including in their development – but is there any sign that the nursing battalions working in the member states are rising to this challenge? The current author's personal observation is that there is little evidence of any nursing presence around the Public Health and Safety Directorate of DG V or in the vicinity of any other significant organisation in the European public health field. Yet nurses should have so much to offer to these exciting new developments. We must all regard it as a challenge to assist and encourage nurse teachers and practitioners throughout the EU to become more involved so that we can all benefit in future from their undoubted knowledge and expertise. How can we help the nursing profession to get stuck into Europe?

REFERENCES

Abel-Smith, B. (1964) *The Hospitals 1800–1948*. London: Heinemann.

Allman, S. (1993) 1993 and beyond. In Quinn, S. and Russell, S. (eds) *Nursing: the European Dimension*. London: Scutari Press.

Birt, C. (1995) *Why Health Should Be on the EU Agenda*. London: European Brief.

Birt, C., Kidd, M. and Peters, G. (1999) Development of primary health care in Russia: public health and cross cultural issues – changing practice in Russia. In *Proceedings of the European Public Health Association Conference in Budapest 1995*. New York: Soros Foundation (in press).

Dainton, C. (1961) *The Story of England's Hospitals*. London: Museum Press.

European Commission (1993) *Commission Communication on the Framework for Action in the Field of Public Health*. COM (93) 559. Brussels: European Commission.

European Commission (1994a) *Communication from the Commission Concerning the Fight Against Cancer in the Context of the Framework for Action in the Field of Public Health*. COM (94) 83. Brussels: European Commission.

European Commission (1994b) *Communication from the Commission Concerning a Community Action Programme on the Prevention of AIDS and Certain Other Communicable Diseases in the Context of the Framework for Action in the Field of Public Health*. COM (94) 413. Brussels: European Commission.

European Commission (1994c) *Communication from the Commission on Community Action in the Field of Drug Dependence*. COM (94) 223. Brussels: European Commission.

European Commission (1994d) *Communication from the Commission Concerning a Programme of Community Action on Health Promotion, Information, Education and Training within the Framework for Action in the Field of Public Health*. COM (94) 202. Brussels: European Commission.

European Commission (1995) *Communication from the Commission Concerning a Community Action Programme on Health Monitoring in the Context of the Framework for Action in the Field of Public Health*. COM (95) 449. Brussels: European Commission.

European Commission (1997) Debate on the Report by the Committee of Inquiry into BSE. Strasbourg, 18 February 1997, available from http://europa.eu.int/wmm/santer/1997/js180297en.html

Evers, G. (1996) The Future Role of Nursing and Nurses in the European Union. Text of a public lecture.

Godfrey, W. (1955) *The English Almshouse*. London: Faber and Faber.

Grand Ducal Regulation (1983) *Duties and Role of the Nurse*, Luxembourg, 20 May.

Hospital Committee of the European Community (1992) *HOPE Ministatistics*. Leuven: Nursing Human Resources.

Quinn, S. (1993) The profession in Europe. In Quinn, S. and Russell, S. (eds) *Nursing: The European Dimension*. London: Scutari Press.

Quinn, S. and Russell, S. (eds) (1993) *Nursing: The European Dimension.* London: Scutari Press.

Royal College of Nursing (1996) *Position Paper on the 1996 Inter-Governmental Conference.* London: RCN.

St Thomas' Hospital (1969) *Historical Note.* London: St Thomas' Hospital

Standing Committee of Nurses of the EC (1992) *Policy Statement.* Brussels: Standing Committee of Nurses of the EC.

Standing Committee of Nurses of the EC (1993a) *The Nurse's Contribution to the Care of the Elderly: A European Perspective.* Brussels: Standing Committee of Nurses of the EC.

Standing Committee of Nurses of the EC (1993b) *The Nurse's Contribution to an EC Public Health Policy.* Brussels: Standing Committee of Nurses of the EC.

Standing Committee of Nurses of the EC (1994) *Public Health after Maastricht.* Brussels: Standing Committee of Nurses of the EC.

Treaty on European Union (1997) *Treaty of Amsterdam.* O.J.E.C., C340.

Weinrich, R. (1993) Germany. In Quinn, S. and Russell, S. (eds) *Nursing: The European Dimension.* London: Scutari Press.

Williams, S. (1996a) Cross-country collaboration, *Nursing Standard* **10**(17): 24–25.

Williams, S. (1996b) The Nursing Agenda for the 1996 Inter-Governmental Conference. *Eurohealth,* 1, 3. London: London School of Economics.

World Health Organisation (1978) *Alma Ata 1978: Primary Health Care.* Geneva: WHO.

World Health Organisation (1985) *Targets for Health for All.* Copenhagen: WHO.

World Health Organisation (1994) *Nursing and Midwifery Country Profiles.* Copenhagen: WHO.

CHAPTER SIX

The impact of health care reforms on nursing – a European perspective

Ainna Fawcett-Henesy

Editors' Introduction

This chapter offers a rare opportunity to examine nursing in some detail in a very wide range of countries across Europe. The way in which the nursing body has responded to health reform in different countries is discussed. Examples are provided of the tremendous innovative capacity demonstrated by the nursing profession in a wide range of situations.

INTRODUCTION

The European Region of the WHO is a large geographical entity stretching from the west coast of Greenland to the Mediterranean region in the south west and the Pacific shores of the Russian Federation in the east. The 51 member states (approximate population 850 million) are often divided into three sub-regions as follows: countries of Central and Eastern Europe (CCEEs; 15 countries); the newly independent states of the former USSR (NISs; 12 countries) and the rest of Europe, loosely termed Western Europe (24 countries).

The Region is characterised by a unique blend of races, religions, languages and cultures. It includes some of the oldest countries of the world as well as the newest, some of the richest and most prosperous nations as well as some of the world's poorer and more deprived countries. Much of this diversity is also reflected in nursing developments in Europe at various levels – policy, practice, education, legislation as well as the public perception of nurses. Nonetheless, firsthand observations of nursing in 38 of the member states, including some of the more remote parts of the Region such as Siberia and the troubled, war-torn area of Bosnia, lead to the overwhelming conclusion that there is an underlying core of broadly similar issues and problems that confront the profession everywhere.

This chapter attempts to analyse the impact of recent health care reforms on nursing from a pan-European perspective. It also describes some of the ways in which nurses have responded to the challenge of changing health care priorities and contributed to national policies and action plans to deliver equitable, accessible and cost-effective health services.

In view of the paucity of published material in the English language on nursing in the wider Europe, much of the substantive material presented in this paper is drawn from the work of the WHO Regional Office for Europe, particularly that of former Regional Nurses Advisors Marie Farrell and Jane Salvage. The analysis is also informed by personal impressions gained from field visits over the past 3 years.

THE CONTEXT FOR NURSING IN EUROPE

Socioeconomic and political context

For most of the past 50 years, the political map of Europe remained virtually unchanged, the various countries pursuing differing yet fairly stable socioeconomic policies. The late 1980s, however, witnessed momentous political changes in the countries of Central and Eastern Europe and in the former USSR. The dismantling of the Soviet system of governance and centrally planned economies unleashed a series of socioeconomic changes, the effects of which are still being felt (Salvage and Heijnen, 1997; WHO Regional Office for Europe, 1997a).

Unemployment and poverty are on the increase in the eastern part of the Region. Civil war and ethnic conflict have resulted in migration and social dislocation on an unprecedented scale, and the presence of large numbers of refugees in crowded inner city areas places additional burdens on scarce resources. Elderly people in these countries have been particularly hard hit by the rampant inflation. Crime and vandalism are major social problems, while fear and depression affect the quality of life of many people.

Countries in the western part of the Region have not escaped unscathed from social changes and the worldwide economic recession.

The core values underpinning the welfare state are being re-examined, and there is growing pressure on governments to cut back on public spending. The implementation of cost containment measures is, however, taking place against a background of rising consumer expectations and demands for high-quality, accessible and accountable public services.

One of the most significant features of modern Europe is its ageing population. Eighteen out of the 20 countries in the world with the highest percentages of older people are in the European Region of the WHO. In the next 30 years, the proportion of people aged over 80 years is set to increase in Europe as a whole, from 22 per cent to over 30 per cent. The emerging demographic pattern has major implications for health and social policy in the Region.

Health in Europe

Recent WHO reports point to the continuing challenges to the population in the European Region (WHO Regional Office for Europe, 1996a, 1997a). The most significant health trend is the growing disparity in life expectancy and mortality between countries in the eastern and western areas. While there has been a steady increase in life expectancy in all countries in Southern, Northern and Western Europe, the average lifespan of people in the Russian Federation and other NISs, has in fact fallen to levels lower than those of 1970. Similar disparities are noted for infant and maternal mortality rates. A mother giving birth in Turkmenistan, for example, has a 15 times higher risk of dying during delivery than a mother in Iceland, and her newborn infant has almost 10 times less of a chance of living until the age of 1 year than has the infant of the Icelandic mother.

Cardiovascular disease is the leading cause of death in the European Region as a whole. Mortality from cardiovascular disease is increasing in most of the CCEEs and NISs and is one of the major reasons for east–west health variations. Cancer is the second leading cause of death in the Region, accounting for 20 per cent of the total. Many types of cancer are related to lifestyle: the higher rates of smoking provide a possible explanation for the increasing rates of lung cancer in the east of the Region.

External causes, such as accidents, homicide and suicide, are the third leading cause of death and the second greatest contributor to the gap in life expectancy at birth between east and west. The greater vulnerability of adults in their thirties and forties to death from these causes has major consequences for families and for economic productivity. An increase in the number of people with mental health problems has also been noted. This is largely attributed to economic insecurity, social dislocation and the psychological ravages of war.

About 12 per cent of the population in the European Region lack access to safe drinking water, and the inadequate provision of sewage treatment facilities in several CCEEs and NISs are a major public health hazard. Infections are widespread, and there has been a notable increase in the incidence of typhoid, cholera and hepatitis A. A serious epidemic of diphtheria in 1994 claimed 50,000 lives in the NISs. Malaria, which had previously been eradicated from all countries, has reappeared in Arzebaijan and Tajikistan, while it has been present in Turkey for some considerable time. The resurgence of tuberculosis is linked to the effects of poverty (poor housing and malnutrition) and HIV infection. Incidence and mortality rates are increasing in many eastern European countries, and the previous downward trend in the West is now becoming slightly reversed as well.

HIV infection is spreading rapidly among injecting drug users in some cities of Belarus, the Russian Federation and the Ukraine, and there has been a sharp rise in the incidence of syphilis in most of the NISs. The lack of sexual health education in schools, the unavailability or high cost of condoms and a marked increase in prostitution have been cited as possible causes for the increased incidence of sexually transmitted diseases and HIV infections in many eastern European countries. The lifting of border controls between east and west presents a serious threat to the health of the entire Region.

Almost all the nations of Europe have failed to address the issue of health inequities within their own boundaries. A 7 year difference in average lifespan between social classes A and E, in western Europe for example, is not uncommon. This is not only reflected in high infant and child mortality, but also persists throughout life for these groups. Substantial health disparities can also be found between occupational groups, the sexes and ethnic groups in all countries in the European Region (WHO Regional Office for Europe, 1994).

The organisation of health care in Europe

Health care systems reflect the overall social and political framework of a country. They are also influenced by the level of scientific and technological development, and economic forces, as well as by cultural beliefs about 'health' and 'illness', 'care' and 'cure'.

Most CCEE and NIS countries inherited the Soviet model of health care, which was dominated by huge expensive hospitals, with many personnel, too-specialised medical care and centralised management. In Western Europe on the other hand, health systems vary widely between countries. In the UK, the NHS provides comprehensive health care for the whole population that is largely free at the point of use. The system is financed mainly from general taxation, and the total funding for the NHS is determined by the government. The private sector amounts to less than 10 per cent of the value of the total budget of the NHS.

In many of the Scandinavian countries as well, the health service is run by the government, in particular by the health authorities at the intermediate level (countries) or the local level (municipalities). In the Mediterranean countries, a large private sector still exists, although several countries are moving towards national health systems financed out of general tax revenues.

However, other countries of Western Europe, for example Austria, Belgium, France, Germany, the Netherlands and Switzerland, are characterised by pluralistic health systems in which policy decisions are made through negotiation between a number of interest groups including health professionals, insurance agencies (sickness funds), consumer groups and government (Dekker and van der Weiss, 1990). Throughout the Region, countries are concerned about finding the right balance between public and private health care provision. Different approaches to the financing of health care systems are also being experimented with.

Current levels of health care expenditure, both in per capita terms and as a percentage of gross domestic product, vary widely between the three sub-regions of WHO Europe. The latest available figures (1993) show that levels of spending are generally higher in Western European countries. However, some CCEE countries, such as Croatia, the Czech Republic and Hungary, spend a greater share of gross domestic product on health care than would be predicted given their level of income.

Although no comparative data are available for the NISs, it is generally believed that public expenditure on health care has declined as a consequence of the deepening economic crisis in these countries.

Health care reforms in Europe

Throughout the European Region, a high value is placed on health. There is widespread support for the Health for All by the Year 2000

Strategy, adopted at the 30th World Health Assembly 1997 (WHO, 1997), and for the primary health care approach. In 1994, the Regional Committee for Europe identified 38 targets (WHO, 1984) with related indicators to support the formulation and implementation of national health policies and to allow comparisons between countries and the monitoring trends.

Health policy in Europe in recent years has been greatly influenced by the spiralling cost of health care. This is largely attributed to the ageing of the population, concomitantly higher levels of chronic illness and disability, the development of health care technology and the availability of new treatments as well as the rising expectations of consumers. In view of the serious challenges to the health of the population (as described above) and the substantial health inequalities within and between countries, there is growing realisation of the need to shift resources from curative to preventive care and from secondary and tertiary care to primary care, in order to change the existing configuration of services to take account of changes in health needs and the adoption of an intersectoral approach to address the 'macro' determinants of health.

A structural overhaul of health care services is now being undertaken in many countries across the Region. Reform strategies are mainly directed at (WHO Regional Office for Europe, 1997b):

- the role of the state and the introduction of market-style incentives to improve the efficiency and quality of health care

- decentralisation, in an effort to secure a better allocation of resources according to need and to involve the community in identifying priorities and making decisions about service delivery

- strengthening the public health infrastructure to promote health, prevent disease and achieve health gain

- changing the patterns of health care organisation and delivery across care settings (hospital, primary, community and home care) to reflect changing health needs as a result of demographic and epidemiological changes as well as to contain overall system costs. Many European countries, particularly in the Western part of the Region, have considered various substitution schemes, for example moving the location of care from hospital into the community, introducing new technologies and shifting the mix of staff and skills, in order to improve clinical outcomes, introduce greater efficiency and the appropriate management of certain diseases and increase patient/client satisfaction.

- a renewed role for primary health care to ensure an integrated approach to the health needs of the individual and the community, and to reinforce the role of the interdisciplinary health team

- developing human resources by identifying appropriate staffing levels and skill mix, and addressing the educational needs of all professional groups.

The need for cost containment on the one hand, and the social demands of the ageing process as well as potential technological advances on the other, create a growing need for the establishment of priorities for health care. It is increasingly being realised that the reorientation of health care systems towards a more economic balance of services can only be accomplished through support and collaboration with all the major partners in health, namely government, statutory health insurance schemes, private health insurers, consumer organisations, employers, trade unions, health professionals and social care organisations.

As a result of a series of major conferences – in Ottawa (Canada, 1986), Adelaide (Australia, 1988), Sundsvall (Sweden, 1991) and Jakarta (Republic of Indonesia, 1997) (see the Appendix at the end of this chapter) – considerable progress has been made in initiating strategies and processes for health promotion and disease prevention. Innovative pilot projects such as 'Healthy Cities' and 'Health Promoting Schools' have been effective in mobilising interest and endeavour in promoting health at a local level.

The Helsinki Conference of ministers of health and of the environment in the European Region 1994 (see Appendix) was significant in stimulating the development of national policies and action plans to ensure a healthy environment as part of health promotion and disease prevention. It also helped to set up a permanent collaborative mechanism between a number of different international agencies including the World Bank, the Organisation for Economic Cooperation and Development (OECD), the European Environment and Health Committee (EEHC) and the UN Environment Programme to tackle the important environmental issues that influence health and the quality of life.

However, the ability of national governments to achieve a sustainable balance between equitable, cost-efficient and universally accessible health care and to maintain steady progress towards the goal of Health for All has been variable. Western European countries such as Germany and the UK have embarked on comprehensive reform programmes. In some of the NISs, on the other hand, there appears to be some uncertainty surrounding how to proceed in the face of severe economic down-turn and the dismantling of the health care systems of the Soviet era.

The Ljubljana Charter (which emerged from the Conference on European Health Care Reforms in 1996; WHO Regional Office for Europe, 1996b) provides a set of guiding principles to direct the reform process and to manage change effectively. The charter emphasises the fundamental values of equity, solidarity and professional ethics, and states quite simply and clearly that the reform process should take account of people's needs, be focused on quality and be orientated towards primary health care. The member states of the WHO European Region have endorsed these principles, but policy-makers recognise the need to adapt and adjust reform mechanisms to fit individual countries' needs and expectations. The importance of clear local policy frameworks and the political will to direct change was also highlighted in the Regional Director's keynote address at the launch of the Nursing Associations Forum in Madrid in November 1996.

Nursing and midwifery in Europe

The European Region's five million nurses and midwives constitute the largest single group of health professionals. However, their influence on health policies and the status accorded to the profession varies widely across Europe. As Salvage (1993, p. 108) states, 'generally speaking, in theory if not in practice, nursing in most of Western Europe is a professional, independent discipline complementary to other professionals in multidisciplinary teams'.

Nursing's purpose is usually stated as helping people to adopt a healthy lifestyle, enabling them to cope with their health problems and caring for people of all ages during illness in ways that promote health and healing, and minimise disability by responding to the direct needs of the individual, family or community (WHO Regional Office for Europe, 1999).

Nurses receive recognition in most of the Nordic countries, the Netherlands and Israel. In the UK, the 1997 NHS White Paper (DoH, 1997) allows nurses to have increased status in primary health care settings both in leading the service and in working in partnership with other professions. Direct access to nurses is being facilitated through legislative change.

In Iceland, independent nurse practitioners providing specialist services as well as general nursing services to a range of client groups in the country are paid for directly from the Social Security Institute.

Spain is one of the Southern European countries where nurses practise with a great deal of autonomy in the areas of health promotion, prevention of disease and accidents and rehabilitation.

The situation in the countries of the former Soviet Union provides a stark contrast. Nurses are usually described as 'middle-level' health workers, who are required by legislation to work as doctors' assistants. Nursing in many of these countries does not enjoy any real status – it is considered to be woman's work and grossly underpaid. Educational resources for nurses in these countries have been conspicuous by their absence. In some countries, nursing schools have been operating until very recently using one textbook written nearly 20 years ago by a doctor. Nursing concepts are virtually unheard of, and the old didactic approach is still considered to be the appropriate way of teaching and learning.

The LEMON Project (Learning Materials on Nursing), initiated by the WHO Regional Office in 1993 to develop with the countries more up-to-date learning materials in their mother tongue, is slowly beginning to reap some rewards. Curricula are being adapted to include nursing concepts, and graduate programmes are being introduced (WHO Regional Office for Europe, 1996a) in line with the new WHO Education Strategy for Nursing and Midwifery (WHO Regional Office for Europe, 1999a).

Nursing leaders in the CCEEs and NISs recognise the need for a strategic approach to nursing development and have begun to formulate national action plans to secure the necessary commitment and resources from their governments. However, the oversupply of doctors, a relic of the Soviet belief in the correlation between the number of doctors and the status of the country, remains a major stumbling block to change. Unless a human resource workforce plan is developed within these countries, there is a real danger that nurses will continue to function as physicians' assistants.

Nursing and health care reforms

Nurses are to be found in every possible health care setting: home, school, workplace, hospital, the community, wherever people are in receipt of long-term or palliative care, in inner cities and in remote rural areas. The major part of almost every country's health care budget is spent on nurses' salaries, and it is into this resource that governments dip when money is in short supply.

As health care reforms become a major priority in nearly all the countries of the WHO European Region, nursing's contribution to the fulfilment of targets has come under closer scrutiny. The five million nurses in Europe are perceived to be representing a major force that can be mobilised to improve the population's health. This is further reinforced in the new WHO European Region's health policy document 'Health21' (WHO Regional Office for Europe, 1999b).

In 1988, the former Regional Adviser for Nursing for WHO Europe, Marie Farrell, masterminded one of the most notable events – the first-ever conference for nursing in Europe in Vienna (WHO Regional Office for Europe, 1989). It was the culmination of extensive consultations with the profession (155,000 nurses in total) over a 3-year period. The conference delegates agreed that 'health was no longer a task for the health services alone and could no longer be achieved solely through national programmes' and pressed for a more proactive role for nurses in the planning and management of health services.

It was at Vienna in 1988 that the concept of the 'Health for All Nurse' as the 'first line of defence' health worker with education commensurate with the responsibilities took shape. The second key issue that emerged from the debate was the need to improve the quality of care by developing more systematic approaches to measuring results. Nurses were urged to employ the most cost-effective measures in their practice as well as to utilise the most appropriate skill mix. Priority areas for future action included:

- the balance of nursing deployment between the hospital and the community
- the appraisal of nursing care for different groups
- efficiency studies of specific nursing activities.

A 6-year plan was developed from the Vienna meeting entitled 'Nursing in Action' (Salvage, 1993), and all the member states were required to draw up action plans for nursing.

Nurse leaders have continued to meet, and each time they have re-affirmed their commitment to the Health for All principles as well as to the Vienna 'Health for All Nurse'.

A final review of the past ten years will take place at the Second WHO Conference on Nursing and Midwifery (in Munich in June 2000).

Capitalising on the reform process

At the Fourth Meeting of European Government Chief Nurses in Glasgow in 1994 (WHO Regional Office for Europe, 1994), the issue of health care reforms was high on the agenda. Particular emphasis was placed on the need for nurse leaders to be active in the policy area and to press for government commitment to:

- equity and social justice, especially for vulnerable groups and those in greatest need
- supporting nurses working in partnership with individuals and communities, and other professionals
- developing national action plans for nursing as part of the health plans
- leading the debate on the efficiency and effectiveness of nursing.

At the Fifth Meeting in Reykjavik, Iceland, in April 1996 (WHO Regional Office for Europe, 1996), nurse leaders with 'fire in their bellies' reiterated their determination to convert rhetoric into action by setting out a clear agenda for nurses. The Statement from Reykjavik included a number of important points.

Community-based health care

Health care systems must focus on society as a whole within specific geographical areas. Needs must be assessed on a population basis and take into account the specific requirements of vulnerable individuals and groups throughout all stages of the lifespan. Special attention must be given to informal carers in order to lessen the extra burden on women.

Focus on primary health care

As front-line professionals, nurses must ensure a balance of care across the whole spectrum of health services, including health promotion and disease prevention. They must encourage self-reliance in health care and work in teams with other health professionals, the staff of other sectors and members of relevant voluntary agencies and special interest groups.

Quality development for outcome orientated care

Care must be patient and client focused, being based on the best available evidence. Appropriate information systems must be in place to enable the use of comparable data on the quality of care developed and delivered.

Competency-based human resources development

Education and training programmes must be responsive to identified population needs and be competency based. Skill mix exercises, in hospital and in the community, must be underpinned by adequate data and focused on issues of long-term cost-effectiveness, rather than short-term cost containment.

Appropriate resource utilisation

The appropriateness of resource utilisation must be scrutinised regularly in relation to its contribution to the improvement of health in society. All mechanisms for efficiency, effectiveness and cost containment must be directly linked with health gain and quality of life.

Nursing's response to the health care reform agenda

The five million nurses and midwives in the European Region represent a major force in reforming health care systems. The primary care agenda is a powerful one, and nurses are well placed to develop a new humanistic health culture that takes account of what people need and want, and which empowers communities to create an environment that promotes health. While doctors have a key role to play in developing primary medical care services, it is nurses, in the true spirit of the Ottawa and Ljubljana Charters, who can turn the agenda around from narrow biomedical determinism to a social view of health, incorporating the principles of equity, cultural sensitivity and self-determination.

A recent project in the Nursing and Midwifery Programme of the WHO Regional Office for Europe has helped to collate numerous examples of new initiatives led by nurses that address substantive elements of health policy. Thirty-one member states participated in the development of the Portfolio of Innovative Practice in Primary Health Care Nursing and Midwifery (WHO Regional Office for Europe, 1999), and the 76 examples included in this document clearly suggest that while the profession's influence in shaping national health strategies may be variable, nursing activity at grass-roots level in many countries is helping to enhance health gain, providing accessible health care that is cost-effective and appropriate, and helping to move traditional hospital-based services into the everyday life of the community.

Among the contributions to the Portfolio is an example from Denmark, where nurses have taken a lead role in the establishment of an outpatient clinic for patients with acute back problems. Nursing interventions in the form of education, information, advice, support and regular contact by telephone enables these patients to continue their treatment and rehabilitation at home. The initiative addresses one of the main health service priorities of reducing waiting lists for hospital care. Evaluations have shown that it also meets patients' expectations of a high-quality, responsive service.

Community nurses face some of the greatest demands for change and innovation as they take up the challenge of providing care to increased numbers of very ill patients across the lifespan. Nurses in Croatia, for example, provide cost-effective home care nursing services to vulnerable and frail elderly people as well as other client groups with short-term convalescent as well as continuing care needs. Elsewhere, as in Hungary, the development of home care nursing services has been supported by continuing education programmes for nurses.

The WHO's global and regional policies for health are underpinned by a strong commitment to safe motherhood and perinatal care. Midwives in many countries are at the forefront of initiatives aimed at ensuring safe and healthy outcomes for pregnancy and providing women and their partners with the requisite level of professional support in acquiring parenting skills. Midwives in Malta, for example, are leading a number of education initiatives in various settings to promote responsible parenthood. Among the targeted groups are men on a drugs rehabilitation programme at the civil prison.

Health visitors in Northern Ireland have linked with general practitioners and mental health teams to improve practice in the detection and management of postnatal depression. Using a standardised instrument, the Edinburgh Postnatal Depression Scale, a screening tool, they are able to detect postnatal depression at an early stage and manage it more effectively with non-directive counselling and listening therapies.

Europe is experiencing the return of communicable diseases such as tuberculosis. In addition, the increase in mental health problems and the AIDS pandemic are creating new demands on health care services. Regional targets to eradicate, eliminate or control selected infectious diseases can only be achieved by the political will of member states and sustained disease surveillance programmes, improved immunisation coverage, targeted health education and multisectoral approaches. Public health nurses in Israel are adopting a number of innovative approaches to ensure improved immunisation coverage of infants born to Bedouin women in the Negev Region and to reduce the spread of AIDS among the Ethiopian community in immigrant absorption centres. Both initiatives rely heavily on support workers from the targeted communities raising awareness of the importance of immunisation, safe sex practices and compliance with health monitoring. Nurses who are involved in these programmes have a sound epidemiological knowledge base as well as the skills to maintain long-term therapeutic and supportive relationships with the target population.

Health promotion and disease prevention lie at the heart of primary health care. Many of the member states of Europe have developed comprehensive health strategies to address priority health targets. In Romania, for example, public health nurses are important members of health care teams carrying out extended screening programmes for cervical cancer. In Britain, nurses, health visitors and midwives are leading various initiatives in the key target areas of cancer prevention, accidents, mental health and sexual health.

In the World Health Report (WHO, 1995), the Director General of the WHO stated in graphic terms that 'the world's most ruthless killer and the greatest cause of suffering... is extreme poverty' and that improving the health of nations depends on 'reducing inequities not only between the rich and poor but between the poor and the poorest of all'.

There is evidence that nurses have taken this message to heart and are helping to address the 'equity gap' in various ways. Community nurses in a number of countries such as Ireland, the UK, Israel and Portugal are collaborating with health professionals, other statutory agencies, voluntary organisations and local communities to open up primary health care services to homeless people, travellers and other groups whose poverty and/or marginal status renders them least able to take advantage of mainstream services.

With the growing realisation that many factors impact upon health and that the nature of such influences is highly variable, the absolute need for a broad intersectoral approach has never been greater. The reform agenda is firmly grounded in the belief that, in order to improve health and the quality of life, health policies must reach beyond the health sector to involve all key stakeholders.

There is substantial evidence of nurses' readiness to work within interdisciplinary and multiagency teams to achieve good outcomes for their patients/clients. The characteristics of good practice distilled from various initiatives include motivated, committed and skilled multidisciplinary teams working towards shared goals, planned approaches to breaking down barriers and 'tribal loyalties', joint education programmes to increase awareness among team members and the mobilisation of community resources to achieve 'health for all'.

Government Chief Nurses of the European Region have repeatedly stressed the urgent need for nurses to have access to appropriate education, training, experience and professional status in order to realise their full potential. The Ljubljana Charter (WHO Regional Office for Europe, 1996b) sets out the need for a vision broader than that of traditional curative care and for proper incentives to encourage health personnel, including nurses, to be more conscious of quality, cost and outcomes of care. The Portfolio of Innovative Practice (WHO Regional Office for Europe, 1999) includes a number of examples of nurses rising to the challenge of creating better, healthier futures by restructuring education programmes to develop the required competences and introducing methodological rigour into traditional nursing practice.

In CCEE and NIS countries such as Tajikistan where nursing has stagnated under the burden of disease-orientated and overmedicalised health services, educational programmes are now under way to create a new generation of nurses capable of taking a more proactive role in meeting national health priorities. New curricula for nurse training programmes in Estonia are supported by the LEMON Project (WHO Regional Office for Europe, 1996c).

Multistaged training programmes have been introduced in Greece to reorientate nurses to the principles of primary health care nursing. Nurse educators are also being trained to support future developments. Elsewhere in Western Europe, nurses are engaged in developing standards or goals and evaluating nursing inputs in terms of outcomes for patients.

Throughout Europe, the need for strong leadership at national level has been identified to support nurses in bringing about change. The 'Orion' leadership programme launched in the Netherlands is an innovative approach to training a new generation of dynamic leaders who can represent the profession in various decision-making forums and improve the public image of nursing generally.

CONCLUSION

Health has become a central political, economic and social issue in the European Region, and there is little doubt that the continuing challenges to the health of the population require new strategic approaches, a strong political will to direct change and the concerted effort of statutory and voluntary agencies as well as local communities. The 'Innovations' project developed by the WHO Nursing Programme (WHO Regional Office for Europe, 1999c) has helped to put the spotlight on the impact of health care reforms on nursing and the profession's response to the emerging agenda.

Notwithstanding the considerable achievements at the sharp end of service delivery, the WHO Nursing and Midwifery Programme is concerned that nurses at policy-making levels have yet to make their mark. A major project is about to be launched to identify with ministers and health planners, nurse leaders and educators, just what the competences should be and how nurses can acquire them. From this work, critical pathways will be developed to assist those nurses who wish to move into policy-making.

As a final point, if nurses are to realise their full potential, they require access to appropriate education, financial rewards commensurate with increased responsibilities, and status that is on par with that of other health professionals. Legislative changes are also a priority if nurses are to respond flexibly to changing health care needs and the rising expectations of patients.

The primary health care approach is the chosen route to achieving health for all. Effective primary health care requires multidisciplinary working as well as multisectoral co-operation. If all the infrastructural supports are in place, nurses could well be the professionals who not only make collaborative practice feasible, but also take key decisions on how patient care and clinical policies are determined, implemented and evaluated.

APPENDIX

- Ottawa charter for health promotion adopted at an international conference on health promotion. 'The move towards a new public health', Ottawa, Canada, 17–21 November 1986.
- Conference statement of the Second International Conference on Health Promotion – The Adelaide recommendations, Adelaide, Australia, 5–9 April 1988. Document WHO/HPR/HEP/95.2. Geneva: WHO.
- Sundsvall statement on supportive environments for health adopted at the Third International Conference on Health Promotion, Sundsvall, Sweden, 9–15 June 1991. Geneva: WHO, 1992.
- The Jakarta declaration on leading health promotion into the 21st century, adopted at the Fourth International Conference on Health

Promotion, Jakarta, Republic of Indonesia, 21–25 July 1997. Document WHO/HPR/HEP/4ICHP/BR/97.4. Geneva: WHO.
● Declaration on action for environment and health in Europe, adopted at the Second European Conference on Environment and Health, Helsinki, Finland, 20–22 June 1994. Copenhagen: WHO Regional Office for Europe, 1994.

REFERENCES

Dekker, E. and van der Weiss, A. (eds) (1990) *Policies for Health in European Countries with Pluralistic Systems.* Copenhagen: WHO Regional Office for Europe.

Department of Health (1997) The New NHS: Modern, Dependable, Designed to Care. London: Stationery Office.

European Conference on Nursing. WHO Regional Office for Europe (1989) Report on a WHO meeting. Vienna, 21–24 June. Copenhagen: WHO Regional Office for Europe.

Fifth Meeting of Government Chief Nurses of the European Region (1996) Reykjavik, Iceland, 11–13 April. Document EUR/ICP/DLVR 96 02 01 01.

Fourth Meeting of European Government Chief Nurses (1994) *Report of a WHO Meeting.* Glasgow, 18–20 October. Document ICP/NURS94 03/MT04.

Salvage, J. (ed.) (1993) *Nursing in Action, Strengthening Nursing and Midwifery to Support Health for All.* WHO Regional Publications, European Series No. 48. Copenhagen: WHO Regional Office for Europe.

Salvage, J. and Heijnen, S. (1997) *Nursing in Europe: A Resource for Better Health.* Copenhagen: WHO Regional Office for Europe.

World Health Organization (1995) *Bridging the Gaps.* Geneva: WHO.

World Health Organization (1997) *Conquering Suffering, Enriching Humanity.* Geneva: WHO.

WHO Regional Office for Europe (1984) *The Health Policy for Europe.* Copenhagen: WHO Regional Office for Europe.

WHO Regional Office for Europe (1994) *The 1993/1994 Health for All Monitoring Report.* WHO Regional Publications, European Series No. 56. Copenhagen: WHO Regional Office for Europe.

WHO Regional Office for Europe (1996a) *Analysis of Current Strategies. Summary.* Copenhagen: WHO Regional Office for Europe.

WHO Regional Office for Europe (1996b) Ljubljana Charter on Reforming Health Care in Europe. Ljubljana, Slovenia, 19 June. Document EUR/ICP/CARE 94 01/CN 01. Rev. 1. Copenhagen: WHO Regional Office for Europe.

WHO Regional Office for Europe (1996c) Learning Materials on Nursing. Document EUR/ICP/DLVR 02/96. Copenhagen: WHO Regional Office for Europe.

WHO Regional Office for Europe (1997a) *The Health Policy for Europe*. Working document for consultation, EUR/ICP/EXCC 010101 – Draft. Copenhagen: WHO Regional Office for Europe.

WHO Regional Office for Europe (1997b) *Analysis of Current Strategies*. WHO Regional Publications, European Series No. 72. Copenhagen: WHO Regional Office for Europe.

WHO Regional Office for Europe (1999a) *'Nurses and Midwives for Health' – a WHO European strategy for nursing and midwifery education*. Ref. DLVR020301. Copenhagen: WHO Regional Office for Europe.

WHO Regional Office for Europe (1999b) Health21 – health for all in the 21st century. European Health for All Series No. 6. Copenhagen: WHO Regional Office for Europe.

WHO Regional Office for Europe (1999c) *Portfolio of Innovative Practice in Primary Health Care Nursing and Midwifery*. Copenhagen: Nursing and Midwifery Programme (in press), WHO Regional Office for Europe.

CHAPTER SEVEN

The European Oncology Nursing Society

Nora Kearney and Kathy Redmond

Editors' Introduction

The context of the chapter is Europe, taking the specific focus of the European Oncology Nursing Society. The role of the society is examined as a major influence on policy development in Europe, the vital role of professional networking being illustrated as part of this process. The model suggests the capacity of nurses to influence policy when sensibly linked and when a clear flow of a specialist service is defined.

INTRODUCTION

As we enter the new millennium, we are faced with ever-changing health care policies that have a direct impact on our health care systems. As a consequence, the delivery of health care, particularly nursing care, in this dynamic environment faces many challenges. These are confounded by the ever-increasing financial constraints imposed by governments on health care spending and the demands by a more knowledgeable public for improved health care services.

Nursing, as the largest group of health professionals in Europe, is not immune to these pressures. Indeed, as a direct result of being the most costly service, nursing has often been at the centre of health care reforms. This is perhaps an acknowledgement of the important contribution that nurses make to health care and the role they have in ensuring the delivery of a cost-efficient service. The awareness of the value of nursing has evolved over the past 20 years, and there is a growing acceptance from both the public and related health care professionals of the potential impact of nursing. Despite this, it has been demonstrated throughout this book that nursing as a profession has not realised its potential at a political level, and we must therefore question how nursing is to secure its future in health care.

This chapter will describe how one organisation, the European Oncology Nursing Society (EONS), has become a major player in the politics of cancer care in the geographical area of Europe.

THE EUROPEAN ONCOLOGY NURSING SOCIETY

The EONS was established in 1984 as a federation of organisations, institutions and agencies supporting nurses in cancer care. At present, the EONS has a membership of over 50 organisations, representing over 15,000 nurses in 25 countries across Europe. The purpose of the Society is to promote and develop cancer nursing throughout Europe to facilitate optimal patient outcomes. This is achieved by a number of activities organised by the Society, some of which will be discussed later in this chapter. The Society has its own secretariat, based in Brussels, and is a full member of the Federation of European Cancer Societies.

Since its inception, the overriding ambition of the Society has been to improve the care of patients with cancer throughout Europe through the medium of nursing care. One could question whether this is necessary, and indeed whether it is the role of nursing to address, in a global fashion, the care – or lack of care – received by individuals in individual countries.

THE BURDEN OF CANCER IN EUROPE

Cancer currently accounts for around a quarter of the overall mortality in most EU countries and, given the increasing ageing population, this figure is likely to increase in the foreseeable future. One in three EU citizens will develop cancer, and one in four will die from the disease (Esteves *et al.*, 1993). Each year, there are 1,300,000 individuals newly diagnosed with cancer and 840,000 deaths related to the disease. This figure, high as it is, represents only a small proportion of the human, social and financial costs that are a direct result of this disease and gives no indication of the number of individuals living with cancer.

Recognising the scale of this disease in Europe, the European Commission, following a meeting of the heads of state and governments, established the 'Europe Against Cancer' programme in 1986. This development benefited from political consensus on the need to accelerate the fight against cancer in the European population (EAC Evaluation Committee, 1992). The initial ambition of the programme was to promote activities on a European scale that would enhance and extend initiatives undertaken within member states (Figure 7.1). In 1986, a committee of cancer experts was formed to advise the European Commission on the scientific content of the programme, and the first action plan was developed for 1987–89. In light of the encouraging results obtained as a result of this programme, the Council of Ministers and the European Parliament approved the implementation of a second action plan for 1990–94. An evaluation of the first 6 years of the programme was approved by the Commission in 1993. This led to the Council's recognition of the importance of the Europe Against Cancer programme and consent to develop the third action plan for the programme. This third action plan, while maintaining continuity of the Europe Against Cancer programme, also took into account other EU activities in the field of public health, particularly those dealt with under Article 129 of the Maastricht Treaty. The third action plan was approved in 1996.

- Data collection and research
- Information and health education
- Early detection and screening
- Training and quality control

Figure 7.1 Europe Against Cancer programme: areas of activity

One of the initial functions of the Europe Against Cancer programme was the production of guidelines aimed at reducing cancer mortality by 15 per cent in the EC by the year 2000. However, the ambitious target of the heads of state in declaring an overall reduction in cancer mortality by 15 per cent is unlikely to be achieved by the year 2000, and nor are the UK targets, which set similar, unrealistic goals. Indeed, if we are to believe authors such as Smith *et al.* (1993) and Beardsley (1994), survival for individuals with cancer has not significantly improved overall in the past 10 years. Given the enormity of the situation and the lack of major improvements in survival rate, it is clear that, for the majority of individuals who develop cancer, there remains a huge issue in relation to providing health care that addresses their needs. In many situations, nurses are in a position to provide much of this care if they are adequately supported to do so.

Whatever is done to address the problem of cancer, from its prevention to the delivery of palliative care, it is the nurse who is the common denominator wherever patients are cared for. Indeed in 1986, the European Commission acknowledged the importance of nursing when it stated:

> Of all health care professionals, it is the nurses who are most frequently in contact with patients. Accordingly, they play an important part in the fight against cancer.

It was recognition of the potential impact of cancer nursing that led to the establishment of EONS as an organisation that could, from a clinical standpoint, address the inadequacies of cancer care across Europe.

HEALTH CARE POLICY

Health care policy throughout Europe is aimed at delivering an efficient and equitable service to individuals requiring health care. In attempting to deliver such a service, there have in recent years been a number of health care reforms within individual member states. For example, in the UK, there is a major governmental initiative to reorganise cancer services (Expert Advisory Group on Cancer, 1995). At a European level, in addition to the development of the Europe Against Cancer programme, the Treaty on European Union (the Maastricht Treaty) has also ensured a heightened awareness of health care policy at both a national and a European level.

The inclusion of Article 129 within the Treaty, while not affecting the way in which individual member states finance or deliver health care, provides the first formal opportunity for the production of public health policies within an organised framework. In addition, the Maastricht Treaty provides health care professionals with a legal structure that can be utilised to demonstrate the contribution that they make to the health of individuals in the EU and, importantly, it affords nurses a legal basis from which to argue for the development of cancer nursing services (Pritchard, 1994).

Since its development, the EONS has been proactive in addressing major concerns of cancer nurses across Europe. These concerns reflect the priorities highlighted by the Europe Against Cancer programme. The importance of the Europe Against Cancer programme to the EONS should not be underestimated. The priorities that the programme has identified over the past 10 years have allowed cancer nurses to focus on areas designated as priorities both at a European level and, through the principle of subsidiarity, within individual member states. Thus cancer nurses, and in particular the EONS, have been able to develop a common strategy for the enhancement of cancer care – specifically cancer nursing – through the mechanism of the Europe Against Cancer programme.

EDUCATIONAL DEVELOPMENTS

The most notable development has arisen from the recognition by the Europe Against Cancer programme of the importance of training of health care personnel in cancer care. In 1989, the European Commission adopted a recommendation concerning the training of health personnel in the area of cancer that included the recommendations of the Advisory Committee on Training for Nurses (ACTN) (EC, 1989).

Following this, the EONS, having identified in association with the ACTN a need for educational programmes in cancer nursing across Europe, was supported by the Europe Against Cancer programme to hold a consensus conference to facilitate the development of a curriculum for cancer nursing education. The result of this conference was the production of a European Core Curriculum for Post-Basic Education for Nurses in Cancer Care (EONS, 1991).

The production of an educational core curriculum provided cancer nurses in all areas with a common language on which to build educational programmes. In developing educational courses, nurses across Europe have been instrumental in raising the profile of cancer nursing both in their own countries and in Europe generally. The curriculum gave nurses at a local level a currency with which to barter for better education for nurses caring for patients with cancer. In addition, it had the effect of harnessing nurses across Europe with a common goal. The pursuit of this goal has consequently further enhanced the EONS, to the mutual benefit of both the Society and its members.

So how does one evaluate such a diverse project and demonstrate an appropriate impact? Evaluation is important not just for the EONS, but also for those involved in the educational developments across Europe.

Many course organisers approached the European Commission's Europe Against Cancer programme for funding to facilitate both the development and running of courses within their own countries. Individuals were successful in their application for funding from the EC because of the ongoing recognition by the Europe Against Cancer programme of the need for the education for nurses involved in cancer care and because of the availability of an educational tool that had been accepted by the Commission. Thus, with the support of the curriculum and an awareness through the EONS of the availability of funding, 34 cancer nursing education courses were, during the second action plan of the Europe Against Cancer programme, developed in 13 different European countries, the vast majority of these being based on the EONS' core curriculum.

An evaluation of these projects has been undertaken (funded by the Europe Against Cancer programme), and the results demonstrate the success of the curriculum across Europe. This has allowed educationalists a framework on which to build their own programmes and has facilitated course participants to improve the care they deliver to patients (Jodrell, 1996).

In addition to the core curriculum, the EONS is also involved with a group from Southampton University, supported by funding from the Europe Against Cancer programme, in the production of distance learning material in cancer prevention. This material is currently being piloted across Europe. The positive outcome of these initiatives has demonstrated that the EONS has the ability to address the cross-cultural difficulties faced by any European organisation. It also clearly demonstrates the existence of a co-ordinated network of cancer nurses in Europe.

This has been recognised by another major player in the field of cancer care, namely the pharmaceutical industry. In recent years, there has been an increasing awareness of the pivotal role that cancer nurses play in ameliorating the distressing symptoms associated with cancer and its treatment. In order to deliver effective cancer care, however, nurses require specialist knowledge. To facilitate improvements in knowledge for cancer nurses and with a substantial educational grant from Smith Kline Beecham Pharmaceuticals, the EONS has produced educational materials on five key areas of cancer nursing care that had been identified as priorities by cancer nurses across Europe. The educational materials were produced following a series of round-table meetings with cancer nursing experts from throughout Europe. The project, known as 'Cancer Care: Priorities for Nurses', has been implemented successfully by EONS members in their own countries, the educational material being translated into a number of languages other than English.

This cascade approach appears to be very successful at a European level in terms of utilising limited resources and ensuring ownership at a local level.

IDENTIFYING OPPORTUNITIES

The development of the Europe Against Cancer programme and the publication of its priorities in each of the three action plans has allowed the EONS to focus on areas for which there are likely to be monies available for research and development. The EONS has been successful in areas such as the mobility of health care professionals and educational development, as discussed above. This success will hopefully encourage more nurses to access the funds, which are available in the third action plan but which are currently under-utilised by nurses.

The EONS has a number of projects ongoing funded by the European Commission, although not all of this funding has come from the Europe Against Cancer programme. The complex nature of health care is reflected in the number of Commission Directorates that deal with different areas related to health care management. As well as funding from DG V, which is responsible for the Europe Against Cancer programme, the EONS has, in collaboration with a number of European partners, been successful in obtaining funding from DG XIII for a pan-European project assessing the utilisation of computer information systems in harmonising cancer nursing practice. The success of these projects has given the EONS the confidence and impetus to move its political agenda forward. The EONS has now established a sound reputation within the EU, and its contribution to cancer care within the EU is now readily acknowledged.

Nursing is officially represented in the European Commission through the ACTN. The committee was established in 1979 with a remit to oversee and make recommendations on all matters relating to training for nurses, with a view to ensuring comparably high standards for nurse education across the EU. (Similar advisory committees exist for doctors, dentists and veterinary surgeons.) Apart from this committee, nurses have no formal mechanism to ensure that their voice is heard within the European Commission.

The need for nurses to have access to the corridors of power has probably never been greater given the major changes that are occurring in the delivery and structure of health care services. Neither has there been a greater opportunity for nurses to exploit their political voice. The availability of MEPs means that all nurses have direct access to politicians functioning on their behalf in the European Parliament. Nursing has a responsibility to move forward at a European level in an attempt to improve standards of nursing throughout Europe, and not be blinkered by the apparent inadequacies perceived within individual countries. The gross disparities in cancer nursing have been identified through the EONS, and work is ongoing to address these discrepancies. What remains apparent is the continuing struggle by many cancer nurses across Europe to achieve recognition as a professional group.

It would seem that, in Europe, we have some way to go before we achieve this status. The recent meeting in Madrid supported by the Standing Committee of Nurses (PCN) of the EU may be a step in the right direction. However, the emergence of specialist nursing groups such as the EONS has much to offer in terms of highlighting the specific needs of nurses working with individuals who require specific nursing care. In recognition of the value of specialist groups, the EONS has been invited to attend, with observer status, the European Commission's Advisory Committee for Cancer Prevention on an ongoing basis. This is the first time that nurses have been represented at this level in the Europe Against Cancer programme and follows concerted lobbying of the Commission and Departments of Health in individual member states.

DEVELOPING ALLIANCES IN EUROPE

The delivery of care to patients with cancer is obviously not the sole province of nursing, however much one could argue the underestimation that is paid to the importance of nursing in this sphere. The complexity of care required by this group of patients demands the availability of a multidisciplinary team in whichever setting the patient receives treatment. The development of any single discipline is, thus, to a varying extent, dependent on its relationship with other disciplines in the field. Multidisciplinary professional groups in health care are not unique to cancer care, but it is in this area that they are perhaps the most developed. The role of cancer nurses in the clinical trial situation and in the provision of palliative cancer care is well documented. What is perhaps less well understood is the role of cancer nursing *per se* and its impact on all patients with cancer and the supportive care provided to family members throughout the illness trajectory by cancer nurses.

The mutual understanding of the complementary roles of different health care professionals in cancer care is vital if we are to advance cancer care. This common goal is addressed through the Federation of European Cancer Societies (FECS), which represents the majority of nurses, basic scientists, medical oncologists, paediatric oncologists and radiotherapists working in cancer care throughout Europe. The aim of FECS is to promote and co-ordinate collaboration between European societies active in the different fields of clinical and experimental oncology and, in furtherance of this aim, the FECS encourages the participation of its members at an intergovernmental level to ensure their contribution to the shaping of health care policy in the area of cancer.

The EONS became a full member of this organisation in 1993. The status of nursing, and as a consequence of cancer nursing, varies greatly throughout Europe, and the fact that a nursing society was accepted as an equal member of a multidisciplinary society sent out a powerful message to European health care professionals. In addition, the EONS' membership of the FECS has resulted in a more collaborative approach to cancer care in Europe through a number of joint initiatives. For example, the EONS has signed an agreement with the European School of Oncology (which traditionally facilitated medical education) to offer educational programmes that are common to all disciplines within cancer care. More recently, the EONS has begun collaborative work with the European Society of Medical Oncology to develop joint educational programmes for nurses and physicians in Central and Eastern Europe. Membership of the FECS also facilitates open communication with a number of other organisations, including the European Cancer Leagues, the European Organisation for Research and Treatment in Cancer and the Organisation of European Cancer Institutes. Such communication ensures that nursing has a voice at an organisational level and is facilitated by the FECS in maintaining a presence among nursing's medical and scientific colleagues.

The critical alliances that the organisation has established in Europe are crucial to any strategic development, and the EONS recognises the need to continue to communicate with all related and interested parties. If the EONS is to represent cancer nurses across Europe, such a collaboration as described above is vital. The need for the organisation to be aware of both political and professional developments is clear, and the need for the organisation to disseminate information to its membership is fundamental to its ongoing development.

THE FUTURE

This is a critical time for the EONS as it has grown rapidly in the past 4 years and has as a consequence raised the profile of cancer nursing in a variety of ways. The continued development of the EONS depends on how it reflects the needs of its members and the impact it can have on improving the care of individuals with cancer across Europe.

One of the most important factors in this is the society's ability to communicate with and to its members. Any European society faces the difficulty of communication because of a lack of a common language. While the official language of the EONS is English, a significant number of nurses in Europe do not speak English, and fewer nurses communicate in written English. The restrictions imposed by this lack of a common language is obvious and at times militates against those who would have much to offer if they were afforded more opportunity to communicate in their own language.

The EONS, as a society, is very sensitive to this and is seeking a number of ways in which to overcome the difficulty. Two major steps were taken in 1996 by the EONS in this area. First, it was successful in obtaining sponsorship from Janssen-Cilag, a pharmaceutical company, to allow over 250 nurses from throughout the world to attend an educational meeting in Milan that was largely conducted in English with simultaneous translation into four other languages. The EONS has also obtained support from another pharmaceutical company, Bristol Myers Squibb, to produce its own newsletter. *Oncology Nurses Today* was launched in October 1996 and is produced quarterly. The newsletter is produced in nine languages, an estimated 25,000 copies being distributed not just in Europe but throughout the world. The ability of the EONS to communicate through the newsletter with individual members is an unprecedented and exciting step. Formerly, the EONS had relied on information being disseminated through oncology nursing societies in individual countries, and while this was very effective in many countries, there were major problems in a number of others. The EONS anticipates that, through the newsletter, the awareness of the functions and abilities of the EONS will be further heightened.

It will remain important for the EONS to continue to establish itself as both a professional and a political voice in cancer nursing. While much has recently been achieved, the future needs of individuals with cancer and indeed those caring for them must be addressed. It will be important to ensure that, at a European level, nurses speak with a common voice in addressing policy-makers.

Collaboration between nurses is paramount in order to demonstrate cohesion within the profession. Nursing groups functioning at a European level have an opportunity to influence policy decisions in relation to health care. We have to pursue this opportunity for the benefit of the patients in our care as well as for the future of our profession.

CONCLUSION

There is no doubt that the care of individuals with cancer in Europe varies greatly and, as a consequence of this, the outcomes for individuals with the disease vary depending on where they live and where they receive treatment. This chapter questioned whether we could improve cancer care across Europe through the medium of nursing.

Despite the historical, political and cultural differences that exist in Europe, the needs of patients with cancer are universal and the principles of cancer nursing extend beyond the boundaries of politics and culture. Shared knowledge and experience can be adapted to local situations, and cultural, political and historical differences can be overcome if a more global approach to cancer nursing is adopted.

It is upon this principle that the EONS bases its future. In harnessing the potential of cancer nurses, we have been able to speak with a unified voice not simply to raise the profile of cancer nursing as a specialty, but, more importantly, also to enhance the lives of individuals with cancer through improved nursing.

REFERENCES

Beardsley, T. (1994) A war not won: trends in cancer epidemiology, *Scientific American* **270**(1):118–26.

Esteves, J., Kricker, J., Ferlay, J. and Parkin, D.M. (1993) *Facts and Figures of Cancer in the European Community*. Lyon: International Agency for Research on Cancer.

Europe Against Cancer Evaluation Committee (1992) *Europe Against Cancer; Evaluation of the first five years 1987–1991*. Brussels: European Commission.

European Commission (1986) *Official Journal of the European Commission*. Decision OJL 346.89/601/EEC. Brussels: European Commission.

European Commission (1989) *Commission recommendation of 8.11.89 concerning the training of health personnel in the matter of cancer*. Brussels: European Commission (89): 1850–final.

European Oncology Nursing Society (1991) *A Core Curriculum for a Post-basic Course in Cancer Nursing*. Brussels: EONS/Europe Against Cancer Programme.

Expert Advisory Group on Cancer (1995) *A Framework for Commissioning Cancer Services*. England: DoH.

Jodrell, N. (1996) An assessment of activities in the area of training in oncology for nurses. Luxembourg: Europe Against Cancer Programme.

Pritchard, A.P. (1994) The Maastricht Treaty: setting a health care agenda for Europe. *European Journal of Cancer Care* **3**: 6–11.

Smith, T., Hulner, B. and Desch, C. (1993) Efficacy and cost-effectiveness of cancer treatment: rational allocation of resources based on decision analysis. *Journal of the National Cancer Institute* **85**: 1460–74.

CHAPTER EIGHT

Nurses influence policy change in nursing education in Canada

Norma Murphy

Editors' Introduction

The chapter describes the implementation of policy and its impact upon the nursing profession in Canada. This is discussed specifically in terms of educational changes and the clarification of standards of care expected. This process of policy implementation is examined within a theoretical model of change. The nursing profession's role as a participant in the change process and as an influence upon it is discussed.

INTRODUCTION

An overview of the Canadian Nurses' Association (CNA) adoption and implementation process for the policy on entry into practice offers an understanding of the role that nurses are able to enact in the formation and implementation of policies shaping the discipline of nursing and health care delivery. Sabatier and Mazmanian's (1980) conceptual framework for policy analysis offers an insight into the structures and processes that influence policy implementation. Through an examination of the adoption and implementation of the CNA's policy on entry into practice between 1980 and 1988, it becomes evident that a framework has been established that could be used by nurses in the formation and implementation of policy. Nursing philosophy and multiple nursing theories provide nurses with the vision and professional knowledge necessary for establishing innovative and progressive practices. The philosophy, in conjunction with the strategic position of the nursing profession within the health care system and a knowledge of policy formation and implementation, enables nurses to fulfil a leadership role in the development of reform in health care delivery. Factors facilitating the CNA's adoption and implementation process for the policy on entry into practice will be examined within this discussion. It is to be hoped that Sabatier and Mazmanian's framework, superimposed on the entry into practice policy, will provide guidelines for nurses as they participate in other policy developments.

FRAME OF REFERENCE

Given the mandate by provincial governments to set educational standards for nurses entering the profession, provincial nurses' associations have established the baccalaureate in nursing as the minimal entry requirement in the future. This shift in requirement came in response to societal needs and the professional leadership of the CNA and member associations. In 1982, the CNA adopted the policy that 'by the year 2000, the minimal educational requirement for entry into the practice of nursing should be the successful completion of a baccalaureate degree in nursing' (CNA, 1982a, p. 1). The 10 provincial and territorial nurses' associations have adopted the same or similar educational requirements, one provincial association identifying the year 2001 as the date for the final implementation of the policy statement (CNA, 1986).

Although educational standards have been set by the CNA and provincial nurses' associations, the implementation of an entry into practice policy falls under the jurisdiction of provincial nurses' associations, provincial governments, nurse employers, university policy-makers, practising nurses, health administrators and nurse educators. Provincial nurses' associations have established Entry into Practice Committees to guide the implementation of the policy, the CNA providing consultation and support. Through consorted efforts, the CNA and its member associations are influencing the establishment of the educational standard, leading to the expansion of baccalaureate education programmes for nurses.

This movement to university preparation for all trainee nurses marks a significant change not only in the education of nurses, but also in the public's perception of the practice of nursing. Challenging this were questions from some of the public and nursing profession focusing on how the changes could be made, the motiva-

tion of policy decision-makers, the actual need for university preparation and the resulting costs to the health and education systems.
Considering the complexity of issues to be addressed in the implementation process and the variety of socioeconomic and political
variables that could impede or facilitate the process, the national
and provincial nurses' associations, between 1980 and 1988, allocated resources to explore issues such as the educational and
employment costs of baccalaureate nurses as well as the importance
of accessibility to the profession. In order to ensure an orderly transition to higher education, professional relationships were developed
to resolve issues critical to the realisation of the policy. A co-
ordinated approach to problem-solving and decision-making
between national and provincial associations, groups within the
profession, associate professionals and politicians enhanced the
implementation of the policy. As solutions to the problems of transition were reached by the many decision-makers involved, another
step was taken in the evolution of nursing education. Issues were
developed conscientiously, while, at the same time, the public, politicians and related decision-makers were educated in the roles and
responsibilities of the professional practitioner in relation to the
changing needs of the Canadian public.

Since the time the CNA membership requested a study of educational requirements for future practice, the adoption and implementation of the policy has been guided by an organised approach.
Although there are many lessons to be learned, the achievements to
date are significant in the development of nursing education in the
country. To illustrate, a new baccalaureate nursing programme was
available at the University of Northern British Columbia in the
autumn of 1993 as well as at Trinity Western University in British
Columbia. The University of Prince Edward Island School of Nursing
began preparing nurses in September 1992. In most provinces, nurse
educators from university and diploma programmes are working
together to plan or deliver baccalaureate nursing programmes. In
Alberta, students were admitted in 1991 to the Edmonton Collaborative Nursing Program, offered jointly by educators from the University
of Alberta and five diploma schools. Similarly, in Manitoba, students
were admitted to a joint baccalaureate programme offered by the
University of Manitoba School of Nursing and the Health Sciences
Center (CNA, 1991a, 1992).

CONCEPTUAL FRAMEWORK FOR POLICY IMPLEMENTATION

Sabatier and Mazmanian (1980), both policy analysts, offer a conceptual framework for policy change proposing structures and processes for the implementation of a policy decision.

The policy framework focuses primarily on the adoption and implementation of traditional regulatory policies in which governmental agencies seek to promote change. Sabatier and Mazmanian contend, however, that the framework also applies to policies affecting educational change. They believe that the policy statement should implicitly identify the problem to be addressed, the objectives to be pursued, a sound rationale for change, and theory to direct implementation. The policy also should provide structures for implementation through the selection of the implementing institutions and the provision of legal and financial resources to those institutions. Sabatier and Mazmanian propose that socioeconomic conditions, as well as the commitment and leadership skills of the individuals implementing the policy, significantly affect the outcome of the process.

In capturing the nature of the implementation process, they emphasise the importance of the legal mechanisms, the dispositions of individuals and groups implementing policy, and the development of consensus between decision-makers. Sabatier and Mazmanian point out that resistance to the policy implementation is determined, in part, by the number of individuals affected by the change, the diversity of their perceptions, the extent of the change required and the socioeconomic and political circumstances. The implementation fails if individuals and groups implementing the policy acquiesce to those who may oppose the policy. To create a balance in the process, the development of consensus between the decision-makers is critical. Therefore, to influence successful implementation, Sabatier and Mazmanian identify six conditions to guide the process. The framework will be discussed using the policy on entry into practice and its implementation in Canada between 1980 and 1988 as a touchstone in an effort to outline for nurses the factors that seem relevant to policy change. Additional information regarding the process is available through the CNA. This chapter does not examine the implementation of the policy by provincial associations, although many of the approaches used by the national and provincial associations are similar.

Although Sabatier and Mazmanian delineate conditions as guidelines for the implementation process, criteria for judging those conditions are not identified. In addition, it must be kept in mind that, although the conditions may be fulfilled, the successful implementation of a policy is not inevitable. Instead, the framework enables one to think about and plan for the implementation process and to gain reassurance on the outcome of a planned change.

Sabatier and Mazmanian believe that the following six conditions are necessary for the effective implementation of a policy:

1. clear and consistent objectives
2. adequate causal theory
3. the implementing process being legally structured to enhance compliance by individuals and groups implementing the policy
4. committed and skilful individuals or groups implementing the policy
5. the support of interest groups and governments
6. changes in socioeconomic conditions.

Notably, the first three conditions are addressed by the initial policy decision, whereas the latter three are largely the product of subsequent political and economic pressures experienced during the implementation process.

Clear and consistent objectives

Sabatier and Mazmanian believe that clear and consistent objectives provide guidelines for the implementation of a policy and a standard for evaluation. With the entry into practice policy, the objective of the policy decision was clearly defined through an examination of the trends and issues by professional nurses. Through the profession's organisational structure for decision-making, members identified their support for the movement to university preparation for neophyte practitioners in 2000. Through the profession's examination of the issue and the agreement of its members at the CNA biennial meeting in 1982, the direction for future education was clearly stated, as were the reasons for the policy decision.

Although the issue of university education for future practice had been debated by nurses for many years, the CNA membership resolved at the 1980 CNA annual meeting and convention that the Canadian Nurses' Association establish as a priority for the next biennium, the development of a statement concerning the minimal educational requirement for entry into the practice of nursing (CNA, 1982b). To study the issue, the Board of Directors appointed a task force representing nursing practice (institutional and community settings), nursing education (diploma and baccalaureate levels), nursing administration and the Canadian public.

The Task Force analysed trends in the health status of individuals, families and communities, the health care delivery system, and nursing practice. Specific trends studied were (CNA, 1986):

- changing illness patterns, concepts of health, health care delivery and health policy
- the explosion of knowledge in the physical, biological and social sciences
- the emphasis on humanising health care and human relationships
- the development of research-based nursing practice
- increasing complex ethical problems in health care
- technological developments.

The examination of needs convinced the Task Force that there were compelling reasons to change the educational requirement for entry into practice. The baccalaureate in nursing was viewed as necessary education to prepare nurses both personally and professionally for the complex clinical judgements of nursing practice.

In February 1982, the Board of Directors unanimously adopted the entry into practice policy. At the CNA biennial meeting in June 1982, the delegates supported this position and directed the CNA to provide consultation to provincial associations in 'assisting diploma and university schools of nursing to work together' towards the goal of baccalaureate preparation for entry into practice by 2000 (CNA, 1982a).

In October 1982, the CNA Ad Hoc Committee on Entry into Practice, composed of nurses from education, administration and practice, was established for the development of a comprehensive national plan to help member associations in the implementation of the policy. In February 1984, the CNA Board accepted the National Implementation Plan for Entry into Practice. The CNA Implementation Plan offered implementation consistency. Using direction provided by the plan and in response to provincial or territorial associations' needs, the CNA developed specific objectives and activities for implementation of the plan on a yearly basis between 1984 and 1988. The CNA objectives aimed to provide support to the member associations in the implementation process and to communicate with key individuals and groups at the national level concerning the process (CNA, 1986). The clarity of the objective, the consistency by the national and provincial associations in adopting the policy, and the development of the National Plan provided a concrete direction in shaping changes in nursing education.

In 1986, as nurses examined educational models for the delivery of programmes, the CNA Board members approved a discussion paper entitled, *Collaboration Between Nurse Educators in the Use of Nursing Education Resources for the Year 2000*. The paper reiterated the clear objective of the policy and the need for educators from diploma and university programmes to collaborate in the development of one educational programme for the basic preparation of nurses. Through the development of a National Plan in 1982, CNA Board members affirmed the intent of the policy by allocating resources for consultation to member associations and emphasising ways in which diploma and university educators could collaborate for the expansion of baccalaureate education. The 1986 decision to approve the discussion paper reaffirmed the CNA Board's commitment to the policy on entry into practice and its National Plan for implementation. The affirmation of support for collaboration between nurses in the development of one level of basic education provided consistency in the implementation process. For example, in Nova Scotia, nurse educators from the Victoria General Hospital, the Halifax Infirmary and Dalhousie University implement a baccalaureate in nursing programme as the one level of nursing education. Their efforts parallel approaches taken in the development of educational models throughout the country.

Adequate causal theory

According to Sabatier and Mazmanian (1980), the causal theory is two-pronged, offering a rationale for change and a theory explaining how the change can be accomplished. They contend that an adequate rationale for a policy reflects the relationship between the proposed change and the amelioration of a problem. The rationale thereby provides justification for change. With the educational policy, the rationale demonstrates the need for change in order to prepare nurses for the fulfilment of their responsibilities in future practice. A comprehensive theory explaining how change may be accomplished facilitates implementation. The national and provincial associations' plans for implementation provide a blueprint for the implementation process.

The reasons for the educational change are grounded in the vision of health care that nurse leaders advocated in order to respond to the needs of Canadians. The CNA and member associations recognised the need to develop health-promotive, community-based services while continuing to provide illness care as being fundamental to the preservation of quality health care services in the county. Within this model of health care delivery, nurses and associate health professionals fulfil innovative roles. The university preparation of nurses, emphasising humanism and scientific knowledge, is fundamental to independent nursing practice within the context of change in health and health care.

The CNA has for decades communicated with health care policy-makers and politicians over reform in the health care delivery system and changes in nursing practice. In 1980, the CNA, in the submission *Putting 'Health' into Health Care* to the Hall Commission on Health Services in Canada, advocated the development of a health care system that offered a continuing improvement of acute care while also initiating programmes promoting primary health care, new points of entry into the system (such as nurses and associate health professionals) and the more efficient use of health personnel. Significantly, the Hall Commission Report to the government supported the CNA proposal for change. Also, in 1984, the CNA successfully lobbied the federal politicians for the inclusion of the 'health care practitioner' amendment to the revised Canada Health Act (CNA, 1984). The Act recognises nurses and associate health professionals as a point of access to the health care system.

The vision of the nursing profession is congruent with visions of health care delivery held by international health care leaders and national politicians. In 1977, the 30th World Health Assembly decided that the main social goal for governments and for the WHO should be 'Health for All by the Year 2000'. In 1978, representatives at the WHO International Conference on Primary Health Care (WHO, 1978) supported the belief that primary health is the key to attaining 'health for all'. In recent years, federal politicians have recognised the need for a broad definition of health, identifying the need for reform of the health care system (Lalonde, 1974; Epp, 1986).

Health professionals, health care policy-makers and politicians have identified the need for the expansion of health promotion and community-based services. The entry into practice policy gains acceptance by members of the nursing profession, health-related groups and politicians because of the soundness of its rationale, the consistent response by the profession in advocated change and the congruence of nurses' vision for change with the future directions of health care in Canada as proposed by policy-makers and political leaders. These variables seem to have been fundamental to the implementation of the policy.

Implementation process legally structured to enhance compliance

Sabatier and Mazmanian (1980) focus on the importance of structuring the implementation process in order to enhance compliance among decision-makers and those affected by the policy. With the policy on entry into practice, the structure and process fundamental to the adoption and implementation of the policy have enhanced consensus between nurses. Although the CNA and its member associations represent all nurses in adopting the policy, there is a percentage of nurses who question the need for the change in basic education. In the implementation of the policy, emphasis was therefore given to the needs and issues of practising nurses, particularly by the provincial nurses' associations.

Legally, the nursing profession in Canada is a self-regulating profession with responsibility for establishing standards for the profession. In adopting the entry into practice policy, members of the national and provincial associations acted according to their professional mandate. As sociologist, Robert Merton (1958), contends, a professional association has a social mandate to provide leadership in setting and establishing standards for professional practice, education and research. The enactment of standards ensure that the public receive quality professional services as well as providing self-regulation, which is a critical aspect of professionalism.

Despite the need to establish standards, the philosophy and objectives of the professional association may generate dissatisfaction within the profession. Merton explicitly acknowledges that changing professional standards may generate opposition and conflict among members and that this conflict is an aspect of professional growth. As stated above, Sabatier and Mazmanian note that those responsible for policy implementation may be tempted to allay tensions generated by change by acquiescing to the opposing forces. With respect to the entry into practice policy, the nurses' associations worked to fulfil the mandate of the policy while recognising the issues of nurses who might oppose changes in the educational preparation of novice nurses. The Board members of national and provincial nurses' associations structured the implementation process to promote the understanding and acceptance of the policy among the members, thereby uniting nurses.

While establishing standards, the professional nurses' associations also responded to the concerns of nurses. Some practising nurses were concerned about the implications of the policy on employment security, and, in response, information was distributed to nurses explaining the intent and meaning of the policy through fact sheets, chapter meetings and other forums. In June 1987, members from the Registered Nurses' Association of British Colombia Entry into Practice Committee and the CNA Entry into Practice Project Co-ordinator met with nurses in 26 communities throughout the province to discuss the policy, its rationale and its implementation process as well as how nurses could improve the availability of post-registered nurse baccalaureate programmes. Similar interpretive sessions were held in Manitoba communities in 1988 in order to provide opportunities for an exchange of ideas and information.

In response to the needs of practice and the increasing emphasis on nursing knowledge for clinical decisions, practising nurses throughout Canada have been interested, particularly over the past decade, in pursuing a university preparation. In the 1970s, three or four university schools of nursing in Canada offered degree programmes for registered nurses. In 1991, every university school of nursing had a programme for registered nurses acknowledging prior learning. Between 1980 and 1990, the enrolment in post-registered nurse programmes increased from 1,913 to 5,524 (CNA, 1991b). Provincial nurses' associations have supported practising nurses in their pursuit of a post-registered nurse baccalaureate education.

Communication between nurses and representatives of the nurses' associations on the meaning of the position, career development and accessibility to baccalaureate programmes has been important in reducing resistance to the implementation of the policy. To emphasise, as Sabatier and Mazmanian point out, resistance to policy implementation is dependent in part on the number of individuals affected by the change, the diversity of their perceptions and the change required. Among professional members, consensus on the policy developed as nurses had the opportunity to communicate and receive accurate information regarding the health care and nursing issues central to the evolution of professional practice. Realising that educational change was aimed at nurses entering the profession for the first time in the year 2000 and that their practice would not be directly affected by the policy, fewer nurses had reasons to oppose the policy. In addition, there was support for practising nurses choosing to pursue higher education in nursing from nurse educators, administrators and representatives of the nurses' unions. As nurses reflected on the professional context of the policy decision, and as efforts were made by educators and administrators to facilitate career development, resistance to the policy waned significantly.

Committed and skilful individuals/groups implementing the policy

Sabatier and Mazmanian view the commitment and leadership skills of the individuals and groups implementing policy as a determining factor in indicating the probability of successful policy implementation. They note that if the individuals responsible for implementation are committed to and motivated by the philosophy and values of the policy they are more likely to make the most of available resources. These authors underscore the importance of the implementers acting with discretion. With the entry into practice policy, implementation was aided by regular communications between the CNA and its member associations. The national and provincial boards used their knowledge and skill to make fundamental decisions about strategy and about using association resources for implementation. Policy implementation was a priority for discussion at the CNA Board meetings between 1983 and 1988.

To facilitate the adoption and implementation processes of the policy, CNA and member associations allocated one staff member each to be responsible for the dissemination of information, the monitoring of issues, the development of plans, dialogue with membership and interest groups, and collaboration with participants in process decisions. The staff members, known as the national and provincial Entry into Practice Counterparts, communicated regarding the decisions and strategies for implementation of the policy. The Counterparts met annually to exchange information, demonstrating persistent interest and commitment to the policy.

Between 1984 and 1988, the CNA Entry into Practice Project Co-ordinator communicated with the Counterparts and other individuals and groups on a regular basis. In fulfilling a central role, she monitored issues and needs relevant to entry into practice and, annually, formulated an implementation plan for CNA Board approval that was implemented by the CNA Co-ordinator. In providing consultation and support to the provincial associations, the activities of the plan provided a structural and communication mechanism for implementation. Throughout the associations' organisation, the policy was made a priority, thereby providing opportunities for its growth and stability.

As Sabatier and Mazmanian note, the consensus necessary for successful implementation requires 'constant and/or periodic infusions of political support to overcome inertia and delay inherent in seeking co-operation' (1980, p. 48). With the entry into practice policy, the focus and resources of the CNA Board members, as well as national and provincial Counterparts, revitalised the ideas and strengthened the profession's commitment to the policy. The CNA Board members reviewed the implementation process on a periodic basis, and the fulfilment of the CNA and member association Entry into Practice Counterparts roles provided consistent support for the policy.

Sabatier and Mazmanian propose that the disposition of the individuals and groups implementing the policy affects successful implementation. Certainly, nurses' steadfast belief that the nursing discipline makes a significant contribution to society was a positive force driving the implementation process. Equally compelling, especially for those responsible for the implementation of the policy, was the conviction that higher education would be required in order to ensure a continuation of the profession's contribution in the health care system. These values generated motivation and persistence.

The leadership of nurses, both individually and in groups, is still vital to the implementation of the policy. Practising nurses, nurse educators and administrators, nurse researchers and nurses within the professional associations have a role to fulfil in this process. Networks of nurses assuming responsibility for fulfilment of the professional mandate help the health professions, employers of nurses, politicians and public identify the vital importance of the entry into practice policy. Nurses' commitment, knowledge and skill continue to promote the implementation of the policy.

Support of interest groups and governments

Sabatier and Mazmanian (1980) emphasise the need to maintain the support of interest groups and governments during the implementation process. With the policy on entry into practice, many key individuals and groups such as administrators and board members of universities and health care institutions, government officials and nurse educators must not only support, but also participate in decisions surrounding the use of resources. Policy critics questioned whether governments and university administrators would endorse the policy. In response, the CNA and its member associations adopted the stance that the nursing profession sets the educational standard for practice and that key individuals and groups collaborate with the profession to enact that standard. Nurses therefore focused on fostering the communication and decision-making required for consensus and implementation rather than on the attainment of a statement of endorsement. Within this framework, information and interpretative sessions were held by nurses' association spokespersons with those involved in implementation. With government officials, sessions examined the policy's rationale, looking at nursing practice and education within the context of health care trends and issues. Government concerns, such as employment implications, the salary differential between diploma and baccalaureate nurses, access to the profession and educational costs, were addressed. In May 1991, the Premier of New Brunswick, the Honourable Frank McKenna, endorsed the policy, stating that the government shared with the nursing profession a vision for reform in health care and the practice of nurses. He stipulated that government representatives would in the future work with the nursing profession for the expansion of baccalaureate education for neophyte practitioners (CNA, 1991b).

Sharing information about the policy rationale and the nature and scope of nursing practice enables nurses, interest groups and associate professionals to understand the relevance of educational change to future nursing practice. Several means of communication were used in order to share knowledge for the development of the change. Information relevant to the implementation of the policy was circulated to nurses and interest groups through the CNA Entry into Practice newsletters on a regular basis. Between 1984 and 1987, 20 speeches on the policy and its implementation were presented by CNA spokespersons to interest groups.

Information was presented to groups such as Canadian Medical Association, the Canadian Public Health Association, the Canadian Physiotherapists Association and the Canadian Hospital Association. The circulation of information reflected a confidence in the policy's significance and an attitude of openness. As individuals and groups learned about the policy, its rationale and implementation process, their acceptance of the policy seemed to be enhanced. As an illustration of this, the members of the Board of the Yarmouth Regional Health Centre in Nova Scotia provided financial support for nurse educators from the institution's nursing programme to enrol in the Dalhousie Master's programme in nursing in preparation for teaching in a baccalaureate programme.

Changes in socioeconomic conditions

Last, Sabatier and Mazmanian (1980) contend that variations in socioeconomic conditions influence the achievement of the objective.

They insist that implementation planning must be flexible and responsive to any variations. Individuals and groups planning and implementing the change must use discretion in judging the potential impact of the variables on the process. In implementing the year 2000 education policy, association board members and the Entry into Practice Counterparts vigilantly monitored and adjusted to socioeconomic and political circumstances, both nationally and provincially.

Sabatier and Mazmanian point out that socioeconomic conditions affect perceptions of the relative importance of the objective of the policy. As health care decision-makers seek a health care system that provides innovative, responsive and cost-effective services, a nursing practice of university-prepared nurses becomes viable. Nurses' emphasis on health-promotive, illness-preventive community-based services, while continuing acute care, could offer cost reductions in health care delivery. Current economic conditions, therefore, may affect favourable policy implementation. As university-prepared nurses are recognised as health professionals, able to provide distinct services affecting health and well-being, the key decision-makers are proving to be willing to invest in the university preparation of professional nurses. The slow and steady progress in the expansion of baccalaureate education could be a consequence of changing perceptions of nursing practice and education requirements.

CONCLUSION

The professional nurses' association serves as an instrument within the structure of society to protect the well-being of the citizens by establishing standards for health care and nursing practice. The members of the organisation, bound by a vision for the future, make policy decisions reflecting the profession's response to the needs of the public. In the case of entry into practice, the decision to adopt the baccalaureate in nursing as the minimum preparation for practice was based on a sound rationale, an implementation plan and consensus between members of the profession. In fulfilling their responsibility to the public, nurses strive to implement the policy through communication and decision-making with key individuals and groups who also hold responsibility in the enactment of the policy. Through sharing fundamental standards, nurses, associate health professionals and politicians are enabled to construct the stage for the future of health care.

Although progressive steps have been taken to define the practice of nursing and educational requirements for the future, many issues must still be addressed in the evolution of nursing. The members of the nursing profession have in recent years gained experiential knowledge about policy adoption and implementation. These insights could be useful as nurses address issues such as the development of PhD nursing programmes, the establishment of graduate education in nursing as the minimum preparation for nurses to serve as points of access to the health care system, the development of community-based multidisciplinary health-promotive services, and the reallocation of funding for the expansion of research-based nursing practice and the development of nursing knowledge.

Once again, nurses need to create the opportunities to bring key decision-makers together and to participate actively in seeking resolutions to issues that build a society valuing the individual's contribution and the sharing of decisions on health and well-being between professions, politicians and citizens. Even as the professional nurses' association has been an instrument for change fostering the values of the discipline, rational decision-making and communication between key decision-makers, nurses must strive to establish structures and processes within the community wholeness based on a sharing of fundamental standards. By actively working to establish the discipline of nursing within a reformed health care system, nurses protect public well-being and enhance the prosperity of citizens.

REFERENCES

Canadian Nurses' Association (1980) *Putting 'health' into health care. Submissions to Health Services Review.* 1979. Ottawa: CNA.
Canadian Nurses' Association (1982a) *CNA Board Members Minutes.* Ottawa: CNA.
Canadian Nurses' Association (1982b) *Entry to the Practice of Nursing: A Background Paper.* Ottawa: CNA.
Canadian Nurses' Association (1984) Canada health act we've won. *Canadian Nurse* **8**(5): 7.
Canadian Nurses' Association (1986) Entry into practice, *Newsletter* **11**(6).
Canadian Nurses' Association (1991a) *Educators* **1**(2).
Canadian Nurses' Association (1991b) *Educfact* **1**(3): 2.
Canadian Nurses' Association (1992) *Educfact* **1**(2):1.
Epp, J. (1986) Achieving health for all: a framework for health promotion. *Health and Welfare* **5**.

Hall, E.M. (1980) Canadian national provincial health program for the 1980's: a commitment for renewal. *Health and Welfare.*

Lalonde, M. (1974) A new perspective of the health of Canadians. A working document. *Information Canada,* pp. 31–3.

Merton, R.K. (1958) The function of the professional association. *American Journal of Nursing* **58**: 50–4.

Sabatier, P.A. (1986) Top down and bottom up approaches to implementation research: a critical analysis and suggested synthesis. *Journal of Public Policy* **6**(1): 21–47.

Sabatier, P. A. and Mazmanian, D. (1980) The implementation of public policy: a framework for analysis. *Policy Studies Journal* **8**: 538–60.

World Health Organisation (1978) *Primary Health Care.* Geneva: WHO.

CHAPTER NINE

A European perspective on the impact of policy on nursing education

Tom Keighley

Editors' Introduction

This chapter examines how the legislation concerning nurse education has influenced the scope and practice of nursing in Europe. Particular emphasis is given to the work patterns of the profession. The Social Chapter is considered in terms of how such international agreements impact upon day-to-day practice, especially in terms of reprofiling the nursing workforce and restricting its educational base.

INTRODUCTION

The history of modern nursing starts not with Nightingale and her post-Crimea battle for the reform of nursing but at a little town called Kaiserswerth in 1836. Here Pastor Fliedner constructed the first of the systematic nurse training systems to emerge in the 19th century. Nightingale visited twice, the second time to undertake the 3-month course. A number of her acolytes as well as nurses from other parts of the world also made the journey to what was a small town on the Rhine, now swallowed up by the city of Düsseldorf. These comments serve both to challenge a UK-focused view of the primacy of Nightingale as the founder of modern nursing and to highlight the European inheritance into which she tapped (Woodham-Smith, 1950).

This history is most important. Fliedner himself was building on the work of Vincent de Paul (later canonised). In the first part of the 17th century in Paris, he was so affronted by the lack of care available to the poor who were sick that he founded the first of the orders of the Sisters of Mercy. They represented a truly Europe-wide nursing workforce by the time Nightingale was trying to put together a team of nurses to go with her to the Crimea. Indeed, the bulk of Nightingale's initial group was a mix of Catholic and Protestant Sisters of Mercy.

From a European perspective, it is interesting that nursing from the 1830s onwards, with the development of religious- and secular-based nurse training, sometimes integrated, sometimes apart, has such implications for the positioning of nursing education and the social status awarded to nurses in different countries. Understanding this goes hand in hand with an appreciation of the history of Europe, especially of how countries came to have their current constituencies and boundaries. In a strange way, this was all resolved by Christmas Day 800 when Charlemagne was crowned Holy Roman Emperor. In another sense, it is still being worked out as the former USSR and Yugoslavia are deconstructed to assume more diverse national and regional entities. Nursing is a part of all that and needs to be considered within such a framework.

This chapter therefore addresses 'a European perspective of the impact of policy on nursing' within that emergent context. A history of major events since 1945 will be described, and the current agenda, particularly of the EU, will be considered, emphasising the significance of this for the UK.

1945–77

Following the Second World War, there were a number of initiatives to create pan-European networks in order to establish professional identities beyond national frontiers (Quinn and Russell, 1993). This was based on the wider political belief expressed so succinctly by Churchill when he said, 'Jaw Jaw was better than War War' (Churchill, 1954). With their usual efficiency, nurses from the five Scandinavian countries had in 1920 formed the Northern Nurses Federation, but it was under the aegis of the ICN that the presidents of 28 national nurses' associations met in London in 1946. Subsequent to that, in 1953, the Western European Nursing Group (GNOE) was formed, consisting of representations from the nursing associations of the Northern Nurses Federation, Belgium, France, the Netherlands and Switzerland. In parallel with this, a working party of the Council of Europe was meeting to discuss the possibility of a common curriculum for the basic education of nurses in the member states.

This dialogue and the work of GNOE were facilitated by the ICN. This provided a central point of contact, which ensured a comprehensiveness of purpose and clarity of direction.

In 1957, shortly after the signing of the Treaty of Rome, a conjunct delegation of the ICN and GNOE met with that component of the EC Commission that was to be responsible for working on Professional Directives. Draft directives for the content of general nursing training were submitted for comment to the European Parliament in 1969 and the Economic and Social Committee in 1970. In 1971, the PCN was established by national nurse associations in Europe and achieved Commission recognition as the official liaison committee for nursing.

This is a key point in the development of European policy and its impact on nursing (Keighley, 1994). The Council of Europe had reported on the proposed content of nurse education in 1967. This had provided the basis for much of the subsequent drafting of the proposed Directive. Council of Europe working parties are government nominated. In contrast, the PCN is the formal representation of the nurse associations. They emerge from different constituencies but have a track record of working in collaboration that depends on an effective national-level dialogue between the two bodies. This is not an issue in the UK, where there is an overlap in the membership and attendance of key committees, shared briefing and a recognition of the benefits to be gained from joint working. It is not the case in every country, especially where the nurse association is weak and or there is a lack of nurse involvement in the government machinery.

Another observation is about time scales. It took 15 years for the Commission to recognise any one committee for liaison purposes and over 20 years to get agreement on the curriculum content of nurse education. This can seem very frustrating to those new to the international arena, but it is commonplace and underlines not the variety of goals but the difference in culture. An example of this is the perception of the UK in Europe. The UK is perceived as being dilatory and nit-picking, constantly seeking derogation where its government thinks that something is not workable. Yet, when it comes to compliance, the UK has a very fair record. The culture of the UK is pragmatic and anti-ideological. In contrast, the commitment to the European goal requires belief and vision over a very long time scale. We are thus labelled by our culture rather than our performance (SODoH, 1995).

From a nursing perspective, the period 1971–77 was a major learning experience. In order to get the Directive that the profession wanted, extensive lobbying was required. This developed the nurse associations' ability to work collaboratively in order to influence the Commission, particularly to get agreement on the length of training. The Directive was finally published in 1977.

1977–96

With the enactment of the Directive on general nurse training, the ACTN was established. This is the only committee that the European Commission (EC) is bound to consult in law about all matters relating to the training of nurses. The structure of this committee makes it a particularly comprehensive resource for the Commission. Each country sends three representatives, one for each of:

- the practising profession
- the educational establishments
- the regulatory body.

This in theory means that each delegation has the opportunity to provide a comprehensive and well-rounded approach to any particular issue. Over time, however, this has proved not to be the case as the level of development of members of some of the delegations varies extensively, as does the effectiveness of the degree of integration that they enjoy as part of their national nursing network.

Despite this weakness, the ACTN has carried out valuable work over time. It has addressed:

- the balance between theory and practice in general nurse training
- the content of psychiatric and paediatric nurse training
- the design of cancer nursing training
- primary health care nursing
- the nursing of elderly people.

It has also undertaken a number of information-gathering exercises to inform its own and the Commission's work. Its future agenda is to address the nature of specialisation in nursing education at both pre- and postregistration levels. This will enable the ACTN to decide whether any further guidance should be issued on these subjects. Given how long it took to get the Directive adopted, what has followed represents an absolute torrent of achievement.

The listing of the work, however, obscures the highly significant developments in the ways of working adopted by the ACTN. To begin with, it is important to consider how the agenda for the ACTN has emerged and with what ends in mind. The ACTN has always been influenced by two major stimuli, the first of which is the overarching agenda for nursing from the PCN. Through the nurse associations, an increasing wish has emerged to influence the European agenda on all issues relating to health and employment. This has been embodied in the work of the PCN. A liaison between the ACTN members and their nurse associations, the overlap in membership between the ACTN and the PCN, and the briefing of ACTN delegations by governments has resulted in a cohesive external agenda. The internal agenda has emerged from the European Commission itself. This has been almost completely focused on the issue of free movement of the workforce. The different imperatives are therefore very clear.

The profession has used the European component of its work as a way of advancing the development of the profession. In consequence, work on paediatric, psychiatric, oncological and gerontological nursing as well as primary care is very important. In contrast, the Commission have only felt duty bound to support work on those issues that would ensure free movement. As a result, fewer Commission resources have been put into the ACTN over time. The number of meetings scheduled and the extent of working group activity have been restricted. Indeed, some of the ACTN's activities have been dependent, fully or in part, on external resources. This has been particularly true in recent years when the rapporteur to any working group has had the onerous task of negotiating with the Commission and seeking external resources where necessary to fulfil the various working groups remits.

No analysis of this part of the agenda would be complete without a consideration of the interests of two other significant bodies. The first is the Council of Europe. Reference has been made to its report on general nurse training in 1967. In 1994, it produced a further report (European Health Committee Working Party on the Role and Education of Nurses, 1994), which has acted as a major stimulus to the European Commission to respond positively to the interest emerging in the ACTN to look at the need to revise the general nursing Directive. The Council of Europe's standing as a governmental body, and its coverage of a much wider Europe than the EU, enables it to act as a major stimulus to, and commentator on, other pan-European organisations.

The second organisation is WHO Europe. Based in Copenhagen, it has been responsible for a number of European-wide initiatives on nursing. These include work on the nursing process, nursing research and nursing leadership. In 1989, WHO Europe issued extremely influential papers on nursing education, practice and research (WHO, 1989), which have acted as a benchmark for much European thinking on these subjects. In recent years, the standing of WHO has enabled work on the development of nursing to occur rapidly in Eastern Europe as the new countries have emerged from behind the Iron Curtain (Salvage and Heijnen, 1997). They have often used the ACTN guidance papers as well as the Directive on general nursing as the framework against which they have restructured their nurse education.

CURRENT AGENDA

With this as backdrop, the current European agenda and its impact on UK nursing becomes more understandable. It can be considered under the following headings:

1. easier forms of free movement
2. common challenges
3. national interests.

While there is some overlap between these divisions, it is helpful to address them singly in order to elucidate the issues.

Free movement

The EU currently consists of 15 countries:

Austria	Ireland	Belgium
Italy	Denmark	Luxembourg
France	Netherlands	Finland
Portugal	Germany	Spain
Greece	Sweden	UK

These countries, as part of their membership of the EU, agree to follow the law and associated Directives of the EU. The countries of the European Economic Area also agree to this in order to enjoy the open trade agreements. These countries are:

Norway	Liechtenstein	Republic of Ireland

This means that 18 countries produce professionals trained or educated to a similar level in order to enable them to enjoy free movement in the practice of their profession. There are currently 13 countries seeking accession to the EU. It is anticipated that several of the countries in central, eastern and southern Europe will have joined the EU by the turn of the century.

This has highly significant implications for nurses:

- There is the opportunity to live and work in an ever-increasing number of European countries, assuming administrative compliance and relevant language skills
- There is a shared training/education base, the opportunity to be part of Socrates and Leonardo programmes, and the inclusion of a European focus on health care or language learning in nurse training
- There is EU wide employee protection at work. This includes health and safety legislation, equal pay provisions, manual handling legislation and sex discrimination case law as well as Directives on maternity leave, working time, rest periods and collective redundancies
- There is co-operation on public health initiatives, including initiatives on cancer and AIDS, and systems for information exchange
- There are minimum standards agreed on food preparation, drug manufacture, water and air quality, and waste disposal, all of which have an effect on the users of health service and on the structure and processes of its provision.

This framework of legislation, combined with the sectoral Directive on general nurse training, provides the context for policy, which influences nursing, as it emerges from Europe. Two other major influences remain to be assessed for their potential future impact. The first is the development of the general system Directives (European Commission, 1989, 1992) and the second the Maastricht Treaty (ECC, 1992).

The general system Directives have arisen from the frustration of getting sectoral Directives agreed for each of the occupational groups. By 1992, sectoral Directives had been agreed for general practitioners, nurses (general care), midwives, veterinary surgeons, dentists and pharmacists. After 17 years, the architects were getting close to agreement! While larger and politically sensitive parts of the workforce could be usefully dealt with through this mechanism, a consensus was emerging that the pursuit of harmonisation that this represented was an unachievable goal. The decision was thus taken in 1988 by the

Council of Ministers to establish a system based on the mutual recognition of professional diplomas through the general system Directives. It would then become the responsibility of the regulatory authorities in each country to determine whether further training and/or experience was required before granting recognition.

This development acknowledged to a degree what was already going on (Ness *et al.*, 1993). By 1992, the second general system had been introduced for pre-diploma level qualifications, notably vocational qualifications, to address the free movement requirements of non-diploma level education. Discussions are currently underway on the possibility of a third general system Directive to provide a mutual recognition system for those not otherwise covered, for example specialist nurses at preregistration level, such as psychiatric nurses. An observation to be made about this series of developments is that it will be some time before its implications can be assessed. A personal view would be that, given the language constraints on free movement, it will be of greater benefit than dis-benefit to the UK when trying to enhance the workforce.

The second major influence is the Maastricht Treaty or, as it is properly known, the Treaty of European Union. The Treaty is important because it:

- introduced the concept of the EU citizen with the right to reside in any member state, vote in their elections, receive diplomatic or consular protection from any member state and to petition the EU Parliament
- extended the powers of the EU Parliament
- tightened financial and budgetary control
- introduced the machinery to determine common policies on foreign and security matters, justice and home affairs
- included a protocol on social policy, which the UK 'opted out' of (but signed in 1997)
- determined a degree of legal competence on public health.

The Treaty also addresses other matters, the two key aspects for nursing being the Social Protocol (Chapter) and the provisions on Public Health (Article 129) amended in the Amsterdam Treaty (Permanent Representatives Committee, 1998) to Article 152.

The Social Chapter was drafted to update the Social Charter agreed in 1989 but which the UK also refused to sign until 1997. The UK government has consistently taken the view that such legislation is an inappropriate intrusion into the sovereignty of the UK and that it reduces the capacity of all countries to operate as economically, efficiently and effectively as they might. This view changed to a certain degree with the election of the Labour government in 1997 on a comparatively pro-European ticket. However, as all the UK's EU trading partners adhere to both the Social Charter and Social Chapter, there was a movement to implement their principles in the UK, simply as a way of maintaining good trading relationships. From an EU perspective, there is clearly a linkage between the Social legislation and the developing Public Health Competency, a relationship between work, social welfare and the health profile of the individual.

Article 129 of the Maastricht Treaty, about which the UK government also had major reservations, lays out some initial expectations, which are of significance for nursing. While health and safety had been part of the Treaty of Rome and subsequent policy initiatives had been launched on the environment, with the express purpose of protecting human health, for example, on cancer and on AIDS, health has been marginal to the EU agenda. Article 129 lays out four principles with the overarching aim of co-ordinating existing and new national health policies by:

- co-ordination aimed at disease prevention through the promotion of research, health information and education
- action in the European Commission to promote such co-ordination
- co-operation with countries outside the EU
- after consulting with the Economic and Social Welfare Committee, adopting incentives to promote public health.

Although hidden in such a summary, a key point in this Article is that all EU policies can now be considered to determine their impact on health. The Framework for Action in the Field of Public Health (CEC, 1993) agreed in 1993 put some flesh on these bones.

Article 152 of the Amsterdam Treaty went further by giving a competency (authority) to the European Commission to become more involved in health. This focuses primarily on aspects of public health. The intention is to make sure that health protection is actively considered when EU policies are being determined and implemented. Several strands of work were identified that would be taken forward in conjunction with national policies in those fields. They include action against major health scourges, promoting research into the causes of ill-health, and generating health information and education. Implementation rests within Directorate F of DG V (Employment, Industrial Relations and Social Affairs). The Committee of Permanent Representatives issued the Future Framework for Action in the Field of Public Health in April 1998. It will require strong leadership to give a real thrust to this work as 18 Directorates General have elements of public health in their remit. Both Articles do, and can, have further impact on the policy framework for nursing in the future.

Common challenges

It is perhaps more readily recognised across Europe than here in these 'off-shore islands' that all developed countries are open and prey to the same challenges, particularly in the economic and human resource areas (Buchan *et al.*, 1992). It is important to appreciate that the slowly decreasing birth rate, the increasing survival rate, especially among older people, and the increasing cost of health and social care are common problems. The size of the challenge suggests that there is a need for rethinking some assumptions. The fall in the number of 16–18-year-olds coming into the workforce not only reduces the tax and/or insurance contribution to health care finance, it also presents major workforce problems as the supply of labour falls in what is, and is likely to remain, a labour-intensive employment area. Equally, while the demand for care from elderly people has shifted back from the 65–75 age group to over-80s, once these people come into the health service, their care is intensive in terms of nursing time and energy (Eurostat, 1988; Nijkamp *et al.*,1991).

This emergent shortage of people is occurring as people's expectations about care are heightened. These expectations are in part fed by technical and pharmacological developments. They are high cost and will, if not in the short term certainly in the next 10–15 years, underline the difference between those who can afford to contribute to their care and those who cannot. This is a distinction that nurses have never been comfortable with, especially in the UK over the past 50 years.

These challenges will lead to the reshaping of the nursing workforce and its education base. The UK has slowly completed the move of all nurse education into universities. It will be in the 21st century that the impact of this strategy on the nursing workforce is fully apparent. However, it does raise the very interesting question across the whole of Europe of who is determining the nature of nurse education. Universities enjoy a very high level of autonomy in every country. In the UK, challenges are already being mounted to the right of the statutory bodies to exercise the degree of influence that they do on course content. The freedom traditionally enjoyed by universities in this respect could have both positive and negative effects. With the rights of recognition available under the general system Directive, one could anticipate recognition of the right to practise resting increasingly on the education qualification rather than on what governments and employers may see as unnecessarily cumbersome and overly protective professional accreditation procedures.

This has been reflected in the appropriately named SLIM (Simpler Legislation in the Internal Market) review (European Commission, 1996). While the value of the general nursing sectoral Directive for the profession has been recognised because of its impact first on achieving common standards of patient care, and second by acting as developmental guidance to those states seeking accession, there is a commitment to seeing how the sectoral Directives can be made part of the general system Directives after 1999. This development, the interest in supporting the vocational qualification systems and the financial and human resource challenges all point to different regulatory and professional frameworks emerging across Europe in the next 10–15 years.

National interests

It seems helpful to conclude this section with what might usefully be described as national or regional perspectives. The UK has had a reputation for being a 'poor' European because of the Conservative administration's approach to negotiation. The permanence of any change of approach by the Labour government has still to be demonstrated. However, as indicated earlier, there are important issues of culture to be considered. One can perceive Europe as being four different areas with different ways of working, and this impacts on the position of nursing in those countries. Northern Europe, which includes Scandinavia, the Netherlands, the UK and the Republic of Ireland, contrasts markedly with the Franco-German countries. The third group is the countries of the Mediterranean littoral, including Portugal, while the fourth group is broadly Eastern Europe. While all of these countries can point to issues in common, these groupings will often explain the way in which agendas are pursued in negotiation.

Turning the microscope round, one can identify marked regionalisation going on in Europe. Sometimes it blazes out, as the conflict in Yugoslavia has; elsewhere, it is a historical longing for separation and independence, as expressed by the Scottish and Welsh Nationalists, and the EU providing the supranational net within which that can be achieved.

In nursing terms, this is played out in the degree of compliance achieved with the general nursing Directive or the other guidance issued by the ACTN. The SLIM report makes some allusion to this. In practical terms, what seems to be happening in countries where a federal state structure exists is that the local governments are seeking to establish separate regulations for nurse training in order to address their own health service and human resource requirements. This tension between the regional exercise of power and national authority plays to the competency of the Commission itself, thus allowing it to pressure other EU institutions (in particular the Council of Ministers) as well as national governments. Nursing has yet truly to exercise itself through this regional machinery, but the development in the federated states may lead to this.

FUTURE IMPACT OF EU POLICY ON NURSING

This chapter reflects on the background and current issues that have influenced policy-making in nursing in the EU. Ludvigsen and Roberts (1996) have prepared a fuller account, which covers all aspects of health care policy. The history is one of emergent structures in nursing sponsored by the nurse associations and collaborated with by the national governments and their international agencies. One can point to numerous occasions on which the profession has influenced thinking about nursing. This continues today with the establishment of a permanent lobby for nursing in Brussels under the aegis of the PCN and serviced by the RCN (RCN, 1996).

The future is much more difficult to predict. Much will depend on the Inter-governmental Conferences and the outcome of the general elections in the countries of the EU. However, one can with some certainty anticipate some movement on the EU regulation of professional education. This may or may not go hand in hand with further work on the specialisation of nursing. Following in the footsteps of the EONS are a number of groups whose interest is the development of nursing practice. The ACTN has already established its interest in responding to this, even if only to issue authoritative guidance rather than drafting Directives. It is within these new relationships between the ACTN and the specialist nurse groups fostered by the PCN that one can anticipate work on specialist nurse education to emerge.

Finally, a recurrent concern has been the level of preparation of nurse teachers. While the move into higher education will lead to one set of solutions emerging on this, the profession will need to develop a view about professional content and status. This obviously relates to the current debate on the nature of nurse specialisation in the future and is an example of how national agenda items often have a significant international component.

In conclusion, it is probably right to observe that there is an increasing interest in all matters European in the UK nursing workforce. This is fuelled by the changes in education opportunities and curriculum design. Given that so many of our challenges are held in common with our EU partners, it behoves us to seek solutions that benefit us all while maximising our national potential. The general and widespread reform of health service delivery and funding across Europe confirms this (Saltman and Figueras, 1997). There is clearly a need to learn from each other, and the EU has the potential to evolve in such a way as to enable this. To do that requires involvement by all relevant parties and shared commitment. The history of nursing in Europe since 1945 is a worked-through example of the challenges and opportunities that such a process generates.

REFERENCES

Buchan J., Seccombe, I. and Ball, J. (1992) *The International Mobility of Nurses – A UK Perspective.* IMS Report No 230. Brighton: University of Sussex.
Commission of the European Communities (CEC) (1993) *Communication on the Framework for Action in the Field of Public Health.* COM (93) 559. Brussels: CEC.
Churchill, W. (1954) Address to a Joint Session of the Senate and Congress, Washington DC, 26 June.
European Commission (1989) Council directive of 21 December 1988. 89/48/EEC. *Official Journal of the European Communities* 32219, 24 January.
European Commission (1992) Council directive of 18 June 1992. 92/51/EEC. *Official Journal of the European Communities* 254209,18 June.
European Commission (1996) *Report for the SLIM Exercise on the Mutual Recognition of Diplomas.* Brussels: European Commission.
European Communities Council (1992) *Treaty of European Union* (Maastricht). Luxembourg: Office of Official Publications of the European Communities.
European Communities Council (1997) *Treaty of Amsterdam Amending the Treaty of European Union, The Treaties Establishing the European Communities and Certain Related Acts.* Luxembourg: Office of Official Publications of the European Communities.
European Conference on Nursing – Report on a WHO meeting (1989) Copenhagen: WHO Regional Office for Europe.
European Health Committee Working Party on the Role and Education of Nurses (1994) *The Role and Education of Nurses.* Strasbourg: Council of Europe.

Eurostat (1988) *Demographic Statistics*, Series 3C. Luxembourg: Office for Official Publications of the European Communities.

Keighley, T. (1994) European nursing – a new perspective. *Journal of Nursing Management* **2**: 293–7.

Ludvigsen, C. and Roberts, K. (1996) *Health Care Policies and Europe*. Oxford: Butterworth Heinemann.

Ness, M., Cutter, J. and Johnson, S. (1993) *Towards a European Market: A Case Study of Nursing*. Leeds: Institute of Nursing, University of Leeds.

Nijkamp, P., Pacolet, J., Spinnewyn, H., Vollering, A. Wilderom, C. and Winters, S. (1991) *Services for the Elderly in Europe: A Cross-National Comparative Study*. Belgium: Commissions of the European Communities, Higher Institute of Labour Studies, Catholic University of Leuven.

Permanent Representatives Committee (1998) *Future Framework for Action in the Field of Public Health*. COM 7630/98. Brussels: European Commission.

Quinn, S. and Russell, S. (1993) *Nursing: The European Dimension*. London: Scutari Press.

Royal College of Nursing (1996) *Making the Most of Europe*. London: RCN .

Saltman, R.B. and Figueras, J. (1997) *European Health Care Reforms: An Analysis of Current Strategies*. European Series, No. 72. Copenhagen: WHO Regional Office for Europe.

Salvage, J. and Heijnen, S. (1997) *Nursing in Europe: A resource for better health*. European Series, No. 74. Copenhagen: WHO Regional Office for Europe.

Scottish Office Department of Health (1995) *Report of the Masterclass on Nursing and Europe*. Edinburgh: SODoH.

Woodham-Smith, C. (1950) *Florence Nightingale 1820–1910*. London: Constable.

CHAPTER TEN

The nursing contribution to health services research and development

Elizabeth Scott

Editors' Introduction

This chapter contains a thoughtful comment on nursing and its contribution to the health services research policy arena. It includes a contemporary history of health services research policy development as well as of how the UK government's concern about nursing has since 1945 led to an investment in research on nursing. The point is made that this research programme is directed by the policy needs of the DoH. The chapter highlights the policy-makers' quest for information to inform health policy. The dominance of the medical profession in competition with nursing for accessing research funds is noted. Details are given of the infrastructure developed by policy-makers in order to support nursing research. Despite all the windows of opportunity, it would appear that nurses have not been able to contribute as they might.

INTRODUCTION

Over the past decade, health services research and development (R&D) has emerged as an important core function of the NHS and is as such a significant policy issue for all those involved in the delivery of health and health care services in the UK. Through the expansion of this field, research-based knowledge has come to form the core of policy initiatives such as clinical audit, clinical effectiveness and patient-centred services. The development of health services R&D has led to:

- an increased number of funding agencies being involved in the field
- an increased level of funding being committed to work identified as R&D

161

- an increasing number of personnel being involved in doing and managing R&D-type activities
- increasing demands for research-based knowledge to inform decision-making at local practice and national policy levels.

The current demands for research-based knowledge to be developed and used within all aspects of health care services mean that the nursing professions, that is, nurses, midwives and health visitors, as the largest professional grouping in the NHS workforce, have had the opportunity to be engaged with all aspects of health services R&D. A superficial review of the current state of play across this field would suggest that, on the continuum of scientific enquiry that extends from research to development, the nursing professions tend to be proportionately more involved in *development*-type activities than with *research*. This has meant that, within the nursing professions, there is a much greater participation with policy developments, issues such as clinical effectiveness, clinical audit and practice development than with research activities. It can be argued that it is in the nature of health services R&D, as an applied scientific discipline, that development should be the predominating aspect of activity, if the overall aim is to achieve a greater use of research-based knowledge in the delivery of health care and services. This line of argument cannot, however, be sustained if one of the key workforces, namely nursing, is not involved or making an appropriate contribution to all aspects of overall activity. The anecdotal explanations most often given for the disproportionately small contribution of the nursing professions to health services research are based on the unequal competition that they have with the medical profession for research resources, given the medical profession's longer traditions in research. It is argued here that such an explanation is too simplistic given the pattern of support from central government that has existed for research in nursing for over 50 years.

HEALTH SERVICES RESEARCH AND DEVELOPMENT

Health services research and development has been defined as:

> the investigation of health needs of the community and the effectiveness of the provision of services to meet those needs. (MRC, 1996)

While this definition embraces a discrete field identified relatively recently, the various component parts are not new. The historical literature on health policy and on the NHS shows that research related to the delivery of health care services has been supported by central government for almost all of the 20th century (Honigsbaum, 1970; Landsborough Thomson, 1973; Austoker and Bryder, 1989). It is also the case that, in one way or another, the central government departments with responsibility for national health policies in the UK have maintained an increasing level of support for investigative research since the Ministry of Health was established in 1919. Today, this programme is provided in England through the DoH in parallel with the support for research provided within the NHS (DoH, 1995).

Research was not a priority identified for the NHS in the original 1948 Act and was, during the first few decades of the NHS, something that was subject to the whim and interests of professional practitioners who carried out their personal research within the environment of the health services. That position was initially formalised when regional health authorities were established and set up locally organised research (LOR) committees with responsibility for administering that part of the budget allocated for research. While the Chief Scientist in the DoH had a responsibility for appointing a representative to each of these committees and for considering their annual reports, these committees had variable constitutions and were susceptible to accusations of nepotism. In 1988, the House of Lords Select Committee on Science and Technology published a report on the organisation of research and development in the field of health care services that was critical of the DoH for the system that allowed it to support a centrally commissioned research programme based on the policy needs of the DoH while the R&D needs of the NHS were not being addressed in a similar systematic way. 'Research for Health', the government's response to these criticisms, was published in 1991 and set out proposals to establish a national R&D programme focused on the needs of the NHS (DoH, 1991). In addition, these proposals provided the catalyst for the development of a majority of the health service R&D activities in the UK.

RESEARCH INTO NURSING

While the origin of the investment in health and health-related research has a long history, it is also the case that the pattern of investment and support from central government for research into nursing has a similarly long record. In 1945, when proposals for the legislative changes were being developed for the new NHS, issues relevant to the nursing professions were identified as a topic for which the Ministry of

Health needed to support investigative research. Amidst all the lobbying that the Ministry received when the NHS Act was being drafted, a number of submissions were made by various health care professional organisations highlighting the need for the Ministry to assume a responsibility for investigating the problems associated with the shortage of nursing staff. The Socialist Medical Association, in a lengthy submission, concluded that:

> The success of the National Health Service will largely depend on the quantity and quality of nurses, who are integral to the health team. (quoted in Scott, 1994)

This view was endorsed by others including Dr Charles (later Lord) Hill of the British Medical Association, but notably not by the professional organisations within nursing (*Sunday Times*, 30 September 1945). The strength of these arguments was recognised and acknowledged by the civil servants in the Ministry, and, as a result, a programme of investigative work was commissioned. The fundamental dependence of the NHS on a trained nursing workforce led to one of the earliest research programmes in nursing and established a pattern of investment that has continued uninterrupted until the present time.

These original research programmes concentrated on two key issues:

- the division of aspects of clinical care that had to be delivered by trained nurses from those which could be carried out by untrained carers[1]
- the retention of trained nurses on the staff of the NHS.[2]

Over time, however, the issues addressed in the government-funded research programme relevant to the nursing professions have increased. The programme now addresses areas concerned with the education and training of nurses, midwives and health visitors, the appropriate skill mix within the human resources required in the NHS and the delivery of a multidisciplinary health care service. The important points here are that this research programme, directed by the policy needs of the DoH rather than the profession's perception of need or priority, has been in existence for over 50 years and was for a significant part of that time the principal source of support for research in the nursing professions in the UK. While the research topics were identified within the health departments, the research was, by and large, initially carried out by experienced researchers who did not necessarily have a professional background. This in effect meant that this programme was to a degree distanced from the professions, and consequently a major part of the body of research-based information on nursing was directed and carried out within a health policy, service delivery context rather than within the profession. The implications of this pattern of development are that a significant part of the body of research-based information and knowledge about nursing in the UK has been developed in a way that has given emphasis to health policy issues rather than what could be described as professional issues.

Within the NHS, as distinct from government health departments, research on issues relevant to the delivery of nursing services has not possessed the same pattern of sustained investment or attention. Prior to the creation of the regional health authority LOR committees, relatively little research was carried out within the NHS of the type that would today be categorised as service delivery, health services or nursing research. That which was carried out was directed by the interest, commitment and grim determination of individual researchers. When research within the NHS was brought into the remit of LOR committees, the investment in research in the NHS undoubtedly increased. That development, however, was not significant for the nursing professions. These committees were dominated by the interests of the members of the committees, who were almost exclusively doctors, and they interpreted the committees' remit as being to provide support for research into clinical medicine rather than to address the locally identified problems in delivering health and health care services.

The nursing professions in research

Whereas research into nursing services has been a longstanding feature of the health-related research funded by central government, the development of an identifiable community of researchers within the nursing professions is a much more recent development. Within nursing, as in the other professional disciplines seeking to develop an expertise in research, early professional developments tended to be dependent on the availability of insightful individuals who were able to grasp and use available opportunities as they arose. There has to date been no comprehensive account of how research has developed within the nursing professions in the UK, although various academic papers have been written about specific individual contributions (Simpson, 1971; Mulhall, 1995). It could be argued that such an assessment would be premature as research has yet to become an integral part of nursing, midwifery and health visiting practice, education and management. Despite this, it can be argued that research in the nursing professions so far has had some distinct direct and indirect advantages, created as a result of the government health departments' need for research-based information on the health service workforce.

Three such advantages can be identified as significant landmarks in the development of a research base in nursing:

- the appointment of a Nursing Officer to the staff of the Ministry of Health with specific responsibilities for research (1963)
- the publication of the Briggs report in 1972 (HMSO, 1972)
- the strategy for research in nursing, midwifery and health visiting (SOHHD, 1991; DoH, 1993a).

THE APPOINTMENT OF A NURSING OFFICER FOR RESEARCH IN THE MINISTRY OF HEALTH

In 1963, Marjorie Simpson was appointed as a Nursing Officer on the staff of the Ministry of Health specifically to advise and assist the civil servants in addressing the problems within the NHS associated with the nursing services. From her position on the staff of the Chief Scientists Office in the Ministry of Health, Simpson was able to argue for, and secure, support for research developments in the nursing professions that extended well beyond that department's usual policies for commissioning and supporting R&D. As the nursing professions did not have a tradition in research and did not have alternative potential sources of support for research-type developments, the support from the health departments was significant and important. While it provided a base on which research experience could be developed, it also provided a model for other funders of health-related research and a statement of the value and relevance of providing support to develop a research capability within the nursing professions. The programme Simpson developed eventually had four component parts:

- a scheme of research training awards for nurses, midwives and health visitors[3]
- an index of research data relevant to the nursing professions[4]
- a commissioned programme of research in nursing[5]
- support for two profession-specific research units.[6]

The details of the programme have been described and discussed else-where (Lelean, 1980). In this context, it is relevant to note that, without the foresight of one nurse who was able to use the opportunities created by the policy priorities of the government department, research in the nursing professions in the UK would not have achieved the position it holds today.

THE BRIGGS REPORT

The publication of the report of the Committee on Nursing, chaired by Lord Briggs, is another noteworthy landmark (HMSO, 1972). The recommendations made in the report extended across all aspects of the professions. The contribution it made to the development of research can be identified in two specific recommendations: changes to the location and structure of nurse education, and the integration of research appreciation into all aspects of professional practice, education and management.

The stimulus that led to the formation of the Briggs Committee in 1970 once again stemmed from concerns over the availability and retention of an appropriately educated nursing workforce to maintain services within the NHS. While the Briggs Committee had strong professional support, it was a government-appointed committee of inquiry, established to address issues relevant to nursing services across the UK. The Committee had a high profile within the nursing professions but also commanded a similar profile across the health care and education services. While it is the case that the government of the day delayed providing the resources to ensure that the recommendations were progressed and implemented, it is also true that the body of support for the report was such that it was politically impossible for the recommendations not to be taken forward. In due course, the necessary legislation was prepared, and the whole structure and focus of education in nursing, midwifery and health visiting changed.

The new system was directed towards providing a more appropriate preparation for professional practitioners who would be capable of being accountable for their own practices and delivering individualised care appropriate to the needs of the users of health care services. This led to the development of nurse education in institutions of higher education and increased the demand for a capability and expertise in research in these new departments of professional education.

As part of their conclusions, the authors of the Briggs report commented that 'nursing must be a research-based profession' (HMSO, 1972, para 726). This statement, made in such a high profile report, was effective in raising the status of discussions on the position of research within nursing. While it can be argued that the statement led to a number of inappropriate expectations of the course and timescale that would be required for nursing to become 'a research-based profession', it is the case that the inclusion of this statement in the Briggs report, did lead to a greater awareness of research and the need for research-mindedness across the three professional groups. The statement also provided an impetus for research into nursing services and for nurse researchers to begin to adopt a more common understanding of the discipline and academic standards required in serious scientific research and development work.

THE REPORT OF THE TASKFORCE ON RESEARCH IN NURSING, MIDWIFERY AND HEALTH VISITING

The Taskforce on Research in Nursing, Midwifery and Health Visiting in England, set up in 1992, was established to consider the position of the nursing professions in the new co-ordinated NHS R&D programme. It represents a third significant landmark and turning point in the further development of professional research. The Taskforce's report was endorsed and agreed by the government of the day and accepted as a central policy statement for England, its ethos being agreed by the other countries of the UK. The members of the Taskforce began their report by adopting the position stated in the WHO Research Strategies for Health, arguing that (DoH, 1993b, para 2.1.1):

> to neglect research in nursing, midwifery and health visiting is to neglect the contribution to health made by these professions.

The Taskforce report presented some 37 recommendations, which were addressed to the DoH, the NHS, the professional and educational organisations and the funders of health services R&D. To this end, the recommendations aimed to ensure that opportunities existed to enable nurses, midwives and health visitors and their interests to be fully integrated into all aspects of the NHS R&D programme and more widely into health and health care R&D.

All of these achievements, that is:

- the investment in research into nursing services
- the appointment of an adviser on research in nursing to the staff of the Ministry and later the Department of Health

- the implementation of the recommendations made in the Briggs report
- the recommendations of the Taskforce on Research in Nursing, Midwifery and Health Visiting

have been possible because of the centrality of the nursing services to the maintenance of a centrally funded NHS. They have been achieved as a result of cases being made within the bureaucracy of the Ministry, and latterly the DoH, by professionals within the organisation being enabled to use the available opportunities in the policy-making machinery to achieve professional development.

THE NHS R&D PROGRAMME

The NHS R&D programme was set up in response to the recommendations made in the Report of the House of Lords Select Committee. It was intended to be a nationally co-ordinated programme directed at addressing the agreed R&D needs of the whole NHS. Introduced in 1991, it has now become an integral part of the NHS, in each of the four countries of the UK, with specific structures and systems for managing the expanding programmes. These systems are directed at managing the co-ordination of:

- the identification of priorities for R&D investment
- the identification and management of a single NHS budget for R&D
- the establishment of an easily accessible system to provide information on current and recent research carried out within the NHS
- the identification and support of specific resources to review and disseminate research-based information
- the provision of support to develop an appropriate R&D workforce within the whole NHS.

While the programme was intended to be co-ordinated in all these activities, it also aimed to be collaborative across all NHS and research interests. The need for the programme to be collaborative has become increasingly important as the R&D needs of the NHS, as opposed to the research interests of NHS staff, have been systematically identified and become the focus of the programme. It has also become evident that the range and scale of the questions that need to be addressed by research are such that they can only be meaningfully addressed through collaboration with all various interests, skills and expertise in the NHS and in the relevant research communities. Furthermore, if research evidence is to be used to inform practice and service delivery, collaboration with practitioners is necessary to ensure that the findings of research are implemented to improve care and services. This means that collaboration is necessary at several levels – with:

- those with the research expertise needed to address the problems, that is, researchers working in academic, independent and charitable research centres as well as within the NHS
- the expanding community involved in commissioning and funding R&D work
- the clinical practitioners who are required to deliver research-based care and services
- those in professional education and training involved in the preparation of present and future practitioners.

THE NURSING PROFESSIONS IN THE NHS R&D PROGRAMME

The main argument of the Taskforce report was that all aspects of this nationally co-ordinated and collaborative R&D programme were relevant to the practice and interests of the nursing professions. The recommendations were accepted nationally, and this provided a broad policy opportunity to enable the scope and scale of research interests within nursing to be developed. The way in which the nursing professions have responded to these opportunities provides a very clear indication of the current state of development of research capability within these professions and the problems confronting the professions in terms of developing a capacity and capability in R&D.

The structures established to identify the needs for R&D were central to all the initiatives set up as part of the NHS R&D programme during its first 5 years. These structures were necessary to introduce a systematic process by which priorities could be identified and new research commissioned. Two distinct structures were established centrally to achieve this objective. These included a total of nine time-limited review groups on specific topics, for example in fields such as mental health and mother and child health, and a steering group to direct an annual rolling programme in the field of health technology assessment. All of these groups had a membership of between 20 and 30 people who were known experts in these fields and came from complementary academic, research and professional backgrounds relevant to the topic under review.

Once appointed, each of these groups employed similar methodologies to reach an agreed list of priorities that could then form the basis of the new programmes of research. This methodology involved commissioning a systematic review to establish the current state of research in the field and an extensive consultation exercise with a wide range of interests appropriate to the specific field. The pool of organisations consulted included professional organisations, academic and research interests in the fields, charitable, and in some instances, commercial research funding organisations and health and social care service managers as well as patient and carer groups. This pool therefore often represented in excess of 200 organisations and/or individuals. The information obtained was collated with the results of the commissioned review, and the opinions of the experts on the review groups, to develop the resulting list of R&D priorities.

In an initial examination of the lists of projects and programmes funded in the first round of commissioning, it would seem that the number of project titles identified as addressing discretely nursing issues were very few and in some instances did not appear at all. In order to understand why such a situation arose, it would be necessary to question the advice given to these various review groups on the nursing professions' perspective on the topic under review. This would include questioning the provision of professional views in the consultation exercises, the input of expert advice on the review groups, the quality of the research proposals submitted in the response to the publication of priorities and the composition of the commissioning groups and their peer review mechanisms.

There is, however, an important and necessary health warning to any such exercise. The nature of nursing and its integration with all health care services means that examining projects with discrete nursing titles does not necessarily provide a complete picture of the scale of work being commissioned to address issues relevant to the nursing professions. Despite this, there is some value in the profession questioning the nature and quality of the contributions being put forward to these multidisciplinary R&D initiatives as it illustrates some of the issues that the nursing professions need to address in order to make full use of the opportunities that exist within this developing field.

It is the case that the lists of organisations consulted in the course of the reviews included all the nursing, midwifery and health visiting professional educational and research organisations, yet remarkably few of them were able to provide a professional perspective on the review topics. One very obvious explanation for the lack of a professional response is the absence of any mechanism within the professional organisations to engage with the wider health services' R&D agenda. It is the case that at least one person from the nursing, midwifery or health visiting professions was appointed to all but one of the nine national review groups and to the Steering Group on Health Technology Assessment. While it might be suggested that there could have been a stronger representation on these review groups, it was difficult when appointing people to these groups to identify those with expertise equivalent to that of the other members of the groups, and with the necessary professional expertise. The current small cohort of research leaders within the nursing professions relates to the stage of development that had been achieved at the time these initiatives were being established and demonstrates just one area of professional need and priority (Lewis and Ritchie, 1995).

When the list of priorities of the various groups was published, several hundred expressions of interest were received from a wide range of different research expertise. The impression gained from the responses received was that while nurses, midwives and health visitors did participate, most were not involved as the lead researcher, and those who did submit proposals were rarely successful. The reason for failure appeared to relate to the research management aspects rather than to the science proposed for the study. A significant number of researchers from the nursing professions may, however, have been daunted by the scale of the competition, and in this instance, it is the reasons for non-participation that are perhaps more important and significant.

CONCLUSION

The case has been argued here and elsewhere, and subsequently accepted at the level of national government, that health services R&D with the single aim of providing research-based knowledge to inform the care and services delivered to the individual users of the health care services is a core activity of the NHS. As it is a key workforce within the NHS, it is recognised that any R&D programme must therefore, as the authors of the Taskforce highlighted, include a nursing dimension. The principal conclusion that can be drawn from this chapter on the nursing contribution of the nursing professions to health services R&D is that, over time, the services contributed to the NHS health care services by nurses, midwives and health visitors have provided a basis for support being provided by central government for their developing a role and expertise in R&D. The crucial role that the nursing services have in the past occupied, and continue to occupy, in health policies and practices provides them with considerable opportunities for developing, strengthening and promoting their contribution to R&D in this field. While the opportunities have been created at the level of national policy, the way in which these opportunities have been used by nursing can be questioned, and in the light of that experience, it must be recognised that the continuation of these opportunities presents responsibilities for these professions to use them well and to develop their own autonomous contribution.

All those who have encountered the NHS R&D programme must acknowledge the current situation in which members of the medical professions hold influential positions in the various parts of that programme and its decision-making structures. The difficulties of competition with this profession, with its longer traditions and expertise in research, are often used as an explanation for the disproportionately small involvement of the nursing professions with the health services research agenda. To follow such a line provides an insufficient and rather simplistic explanation. In the Taskforce report, the point was made that nurses, midwives and health visitors ask questions different from those of their medical and other health care provider colleagues within that R&D agenda, and their perspective is both relevant and important. While the principle of that position has been accepted within government and within the NHS, there is a need to consider whether the nursing professions are sufficiently well organised in terms of R&D, with an appropriate research culture and adequate infrastructure, to enable them to promote their own perspectives on the R&D agenda and to respond to all the available opportunities.

NOTES

1. H.A. Goddard was commissioned during the late 1950s by the Nuffield Provincial Hospital Trust, with funding from the Ministry of Health, to carry out a study of the work carried out by nurses in hospital wards. This study involved a thorough task analysis of nursing work. It provided a detailed account of the range of tasks undertaken by nurses and led to a number of publications, for example *Work Measurement as a Basis for Calculating Nursing Establishment* (Leeds Regional Hospital Board, 1963).

2 I.E.P. Menzies, a clinical psychologist working at the Tavistock Institute, London, was commissioned to investigate the reasons for the high attrition rate from nurse training during the 1950s. In this work, she investigated the stresses and tensions that nurses experienced during training. This was a seminal research study that still has relevance today. It was reported in

several papers including 'A case study in the functioning of social systems as a defence against anxiety' (1960) *Human Relations*, 13(2).

3. A scheme of research training awards was established in the DHSS in 1968 with the explicit aim of providing support to members of the nursing professions who wished to develop an expertise in research. The scheme continued until 1995, when the awards were incorporated into the schemes of support provided through the Regional Offices of the NHS Executive. This scheme was the major source of support for nurses studying for research degrees.

4. The *Index of Nursing Research* was established within the DHSS and provided the first database of research studies on nursing carried out by nurses, midwives and health visitors. The Index, and the quarterly publication *Nursing Research Abstracts*, existed for 25 years and was ultimately incorporated into the DoH database.

5. The DHSS-commissioned programme about nursing began with the studies identified in Note 1; however, it was significantly expanded when the DHSS provided funding to the RCN to undertake a series of projects under the heading *The study of nursing care*. The programme was subsequently expanded to involve a wide range of research topics, research expertise and research bases.

6. With the explicit aim of improving the quality of research work in nursing, the DHSS did, for a time, provide funding to support two profession-specific research units, one for education and the other for practice. These were part of a cohort of research units funded and managed by the DHSS.

REFERENCES

Austoker, J. and Bryder, L. (eds) (1989) *Historical Perspectives on the Role of the MRC*. Oxford: Oxford University Press.

Department of Health (1991) *Research for Health: A Research and Development Strategy for the NHS*. London: HMSO.

Department of Health (1993a) *Research for Health*. London: HMSO.

Department of Health (1993b) *Report of the Taskforce on a Strategy for Research in Nursing, Midwifery and Health Visiting*. London: HMSO.

Department of Health (1995) *Centrally Commissioned Programme*. London: HMSO.

HMSO (1972) *Report of the Committee on Nursing (Briggs Report)*. London: HMSO.

Honigsbaum, F. (1970) *The Struggle for the Ministry of Health*, Occasional Papers on Social Administration No. 37. London: G. Bell.

House of Lords Select Committee on Science and Technology (1988) *Priorities in Medical Research*. London: HMSO.

Landsborough Thomson, A. (1973) *Half a Century of Medical Research: Origins and Policy of MRC*. London: HMSO.

Lelean, S. R.(1980) Research in nursing: An Overview of DHSS initiatives in developing research in nursing. Parts 1 & 2 *Nursing Times* **76**(2): 5–8; **76**(3): 9–12.

Lewis, J. and Ritchie, J. (1995) *Advancing Research: Research Workforce Capacity in Health and Social Care.* London: SCPR.

Medical Research Council (1996) *MRC Handbook 1995/96.* London: MRC.

Mulhall, A. (1995) Nursing research: what difference does it make. *Journal of Advanced Nursing* **21**: 576–83.

Scott, E. J. C. (1994) The Influence of the Staff of the Ministry of Health on Policies for Nursing 1919–1968. Unpublished PhD thesis, London School of Economics.

Scottish Office Home and Health Department (1991) *A Strategy for Nursing Research in Scotland.* Edinburgh: SOHHD

Simpson, H. M. (1971) *Research into Nursing Problems.* Portfolio for Health, 1. Oxford: Oxford University Press and Nuffield Provincial Hospital Trust.

CHAPTER ELEVEN

Of rites, research and reforms: a systems perspective on the maintenance of clinical nursing rituals

Carolyn Hicks

Editors' Introduction

This chapter is concerned with the role of nursing in the development of a research culture within the NHS. The growth of evidence-based medicine in the medical profession is contrasted with the situation in nursing, and indeed the whole philosophy of evidence-based medicine is questioned in the context of the holistic qualitative orientation of the nursing profession. Difficulties in changing the research culture appear to stem from changes to the nursing role, access to appropriate resources and the profession's own identity in relation to doctors and to the nature of scientific enquiry.

INTRODUCTION

The case for research-based health care has been convincingly made, yet the evidence suggests that much clinical nursing remains firmly rooted in traditional practices. In a culture of personal accountability, the temptation has been to apportion responsibility for this to the individual nurse. This chapter considers an alternative perspective implicating both the reforms to the NHS generally and those which were intended to enhance the professional status of nursing, many of which have had a counterproductive impact on the integration of research with practice.

The past decade has witnessed increasing pressure on health care professionals to ensure that their clinical practice can be justified by scientifically derived research evidence (Peckham, 1991). This imperative contrasts with the tradition and culture of health care generally, and nursing in particular, in which intuition and historical precedent have dominated clinical decision-making. The arguments in favour of the shift to evidence-driven nursing practice are powerful, being focused principally around the fact that the demand for health care far exceeds supply, not only in the UK, but also globally. This problem is further exacerbated by swingeing resource restrictions, which create the need for demonstrable cost-effectiveness. Pressure for greater objectivity in health care planning, the rapid progress made by medicine and technology, and the philosophy that defines patients as service users with the rights of consumers or clients have together created a requirement for quality assurance systems and accountability structures, in which research has a vital role to play. Within this context, nursing, like other health care professions, has been subject to explicit demands to ensure that clinical practice accords with the best available knowledge. It is hardly surprising, then, that an evidence-based care culture is being promoted as the panacea to the various challenges posed by evolving systems and services.

THE NEED TO PROFESSIONALISE NURSING

While these arguments derive from the wider health care context, recent developments within nursing have created their own momentum for research. For too long seen as handmaidens of the doctor, nurses are now demanding equivalent professional rights and status as independent health carers with a complementary role. For many, both within and outside the profession, this bid for autonomy is not only overdue, but also deserved, and support for the initiative has been considerable. Consequently, the status of nursing, both current and aspired, has been the focus of much debate, arguments centring on the imperative for nursing to control its own work, to realise its unique role in the health care system and to shed the constraints of managerialism and bureaucracy so that autonomous, professional practice can become the new norm (Davies, 1995). To achieve professional status, however, the core defining criteria of intellectualism – the possession of an esoteric body of scientifically founded knowledge, and the self-regulation of membership and training – must be met. In order to satisfy these essential prerequisites of professional status, nursing has been keen to develop the power of its own statutory bodies, to reform education and training, and to create a corpus of nursing-specific research knowledge that will inform both education and practice. It might thus have been predicted that general health policy reforms, together with nursing's demand for enhanced professionalism, should offer reciprocal support to ensure a heightened profile of nursing research within clinical practice.

Rather surprisingly, there is a significant body of evidence to suggest that, despite these important sea changes, nursing remains firmly grounded in ritual and tradition. In cogent reviews of the area, Walsh and Ford (1992) and Ford and Walsh (1995) suggest that nursing practice continues to be driven by precedent and supposition rather than by rational action and research, and the authors offer numerous examples of ritualistic practices that persist, even in the face of overwhelming counterevidence. For example, blood pressure monitoring is enshrined within the routine of most hospitals despite the fact that on some wards it uses the equivalent of half the working hours of a full-time nurse and is of limited reliability and value.

If the contention that dysfunctional rituals persist is a valid one, it is reasonable to enquire why mechanistic practices continue to dominate clinical nursing care. Such is the concern with this question that a significant amount of time and attention has been devoted to identifying the sources of the problem as a first stage in remedying the situation, for example (Hicks, 1995). The literature in this area is extensive, and a review beyond the scope of this paper, but it would generally appear that it is the individual nurse who has been held responsible for retaining traditional practices (Hunt, 1987), while contextual and policy influences have been largely ignored. Allegations of diffidence, preference for subordination, scepticism and the like have all located culpability at the individual level, while overlooking the inadequacies of the system within which nursing operates. As Salvage (1985, p. 84) notes:

> Instead of looking at the structure and its dynamics to understand and solve problems, the individual nurse at all levels of the hierarchy is blamed for her shortcomings.

It is easy to apportion blame to the individual nurse, if for no other reason than that it allows managers and policy-makers to abrogate responsibility for ensuring that clinical care is informed by research evidence. While it is undoubtedly the case that many nurses do not see research-based care as being central to their job and will therefore resist the pressure to change their established practices (Hicks *et al.*, 1996), some of the reforms of the past decade, to the health service in general and nursing in particular, have impeded the introduction of evidence-based clinical practice by creating obstacles that uniquely affect nursing. Of special relevance to the present chapter are the strategies adopted in the move towards the enhanced professionalisation of nursing, which should have created a *milieu* in which research could thrive. Instead, the reforms to training and practice, ostensibly so compatible with the development of evidence-based clinical practice, have inadvertently served to retrench nursing in its historical rituals.

It should also be noted that the propensity to blame the individual nurse for the persistence of mechanistic care procedures has had the additional effect of confirming the stereotype of the nurse as submissive and reactionary, which is a position consistent with the wider bureaucratic framework of the NHS. Maintaining the established power relationships in this way is entirely functional to the management and control of the nursing workforce in a time of turbulence and fundamental health care reform and is an issue that will be returned to later in this chapter. It should be noted that a fuller discussion of these core issues appears elsewhere (Hicks, 1998a, 1998b).

THE HISTORY AND TRADITION OF NURSING

The historical legacy that defines nursing as an extension of the female role – compliant, reactive, sanitised and submissive – has been well documented (see, for example, Garmarnikov, 1978; Davies, 1995). Indeed, as Florence Nightingale herself observed, 'to be a good nurse, one must first be a good woman' (Nightingale, 1881, quoted by Gamarnikov, 1978, p. 115), thereby ensuring that the nurse was socialised into a subservient position within the hospital, responsive to the needs of the superior (male) doctor.

This stereotype has shifted somewhat over the past century, but not sufficiently for nursing to jettison its gender associations, which cling tenaciously to the profession (Davies, 1995). In a North American study, Kaler *et al.* (1989) found that the public's view of the nurse was almost synonymous with that of the female archetype, a perspective similarly held by nurses themselves in a British study (Hicks, 1996). Given that professions dominated by women are characterised by high vocation/low status and a propensity to adhere to outmoded practices (Speedy, 1991), the perpetuation of the female stereotype of nursing will inevitably be unhelpful in the transition from mechanistic, unthinking care-giving to a proactive and scientifically founded *profession*. The situation, however, is particularly exacerbated by the fact that science and research are imbued with masculine connotations. There is a significant body of evidence suggesting that, even in primary school, boys are assumed to be better at maths, science and technology, while girls are considered superior in linguistic activities, arts and humanities (see, for example, Archer, 1992). These assumptions continue to gather momentum both through secondary and tertiary education and occupational choice, the result being that careers become heavily gendered – with all the values and qualities that this confers.

This gender stereotypy has a direct analogy with nursing and the scientifically based care culture. Nursing, with its female associations and its emphasis on practicality and reactivity, care and intuition, subjectivity and experiential decision-making, would appear to be incompatible with the protocols of masculinised, formal scientific procedures that value objectivity, distance, proactivity, abstraction and the mastery of esoteric skills and procedures. It is perhaps worth noting that medicine has, in contrast, a masculine tradition, a scientifically founded training and a position in the health care hierarchy that grants it automatic supremacy and autonomy. It is small wonder, then, that it has made more progress towards research-founded care (see, for example, Ellis *et al.*, 1995).

Nursing, in comparison, appears doubly disadvantaged: the new evidence-based care culture not only demands that nursing abandon many of the gendered attributes that have defined and dictated its nature for more than a century, but also requires the workforce to acquire a set of skills in which women have been conditioned to believe themselves inferior. This contention gains empirical support from a study by Hicks (1992), which was concerned to establish nurses' perceptions of nursing research. Not only was nursing research undervalued relative to comparable medical research, but moreover, those areas that received particularly poor ratings were exactly those traditionally construed as the domain of men – scientific design and statistical analysis.

Thus the demand for evidence-based clinical nursing is also a demand to reject the gendered traditions and culture of nursing and to acquire a set of skills in which women have been thought to be substandard. The new scientific culture, still in its neophytic stage, is no match for a century of conditioning and stereotyping. To expect nursing to abandon its values and principles in a decade is to ask too much too soon; it is also perhaps to make the wrong demand.

THE CHANGES IN NURSING IDEOLOGY

One of the criteria of professional status is the possession of a specific body of scientific knowledge that is particular to the group concerned. It is widely accepted that, until relatively recently, nursing had borrowed much of its knowledge base from allied disciplines and thus lacked the essential corpus of information that would have distinguished it as a separate profession. As one means by which it could rectify this, nursing adopted a model of care that was novel and specific, one which changed the emphasis from task-based to holistic care. To support this innovation, research that affirmed the worth of this model was required. It would, therefore, be predicted that the new philosophy of care should have spawned a significant output of research findings that would not only confirm the value of the nursing process, but also be a useful contributor towards evidence-based clinical practice.

There is considerable evidence to suggest that these predictions have not yet materialised (Smith, 1994; Hicks, 1995), one reason for this perhaps relating to the definition of research in this context. Although there are numerous research methodologies, there is an unspoken assumption within health care that only the scientific method (particularly the randomised controlled trial; RCT) has any validity. As May (1997, p. 22) notes:

> evidence gained in other ways is [considered] worthless, or of lesser significance, which means that issues not amenable to the RCT approach run the risk of falling by the wayside.

Hypothesis testing and experimentation are easily imposed upon specific, identifiable nursing tasks but have limited compatibility with an holistic approach to nursing care. The nursing process involves the nurse and patient in a dynamic interrelationship founded on 'tacit nursing knowledge' (Meerabeau, 1992) and consequently defies the excessive quantification and reductionism demanded by the formal scientific methods. As Waerness (1992) comments, caring work cannot be entirely contained within and governed by scientific knowledge. If it is acknowledged that care-giving involves emotion, commitment, flexibility and adaptability, it follows axiomatically that the rigidity and predictability that are the hallmarks of formal science have a questionable legitimacy within nursing. To professionalise nursing is therefore to replace the values of caring with those of science. Waerness (1992, p. 224) notes that:

nursing science is... not a solution to the problems of strengthening the values inherent in the rationality of caring, at least as long as this science is based in the generally accepted notions of scientific knowledge and learning.

A more appropriate model for investigating much of the nursing process is the qualitative approach, which unfortunately does not enjoy the same kudos as the experimental method (May, 1997). This prejudice potentially disadvantages applications for research funding and publication of studies that employ a qualitative methodology (Hicks and Hennessy, 1997), yet the dissemination and implementation of empirical evidence self-evidently relies upon the publication of relevant research. Ironically, the nursing process, which was intended to enhance professional autonomy through the creation of an exclusive care model, may in fact have made the *scientific* knowledge base on which professional status depends more difficult to achieve, simply because the model is not amenable to the type of research scrutiny preferred by the new health care culture.

The problem of the nursing process model, however, goes beyond its incompatibility with the hypothetico-deductive model. Nursing is inherently stressful and anxiety provoking, focusing as it does on human distress and pain. The task-orientated approach to nursing, although depersonalising to the patient, at least afforded the nurse the opportunity for emotional detachment and the psychological protection that was consequent upon it (Menzies, 1970). In contrast, the nursing process conceives of the patient as a whole and sentient being who combines thought and emotion, and with whom the potential for attachment is considerable. Inevitably, where there is involvement with the patient, so too there is burn-out and anxiety.

The psychological literature abounds with evidence to suggest that excessive stress or perceived threat leads to regressive and well-learned behaviour patterns. Translated into a nursing context, the irony is clear; the nursing process both resists investigation by the highly prized scientific protocols and also encourages nurses to retreat to the rituals that evidence-based care was intended to counteract. In its desire to achieve the esoteric body of scientific knowledge required for professional status, nursing has inadvertently made its acquisition more difficult.

CHANGES IN EDUCATION AND TRAINING

The implementation of the strategy Project 2000 for the reform of basic nurse education forged an inextricable link between nurse training and the higher education sector. The objective of this merger was the need for an academic education for nurses rather than a vocational apprenticeship, this being one criterion of professional status. Part of the merger process inevitably involved the assimilation of the values and ideals espoused by the host institution. Since research is a core activity of universities, one product of nursing's new relationship with higher education might logically be expected to be an increase in research activity. This outcome should have been further facilitated by the fact that, for more than a decade, university funding allocations have been determined by research productivity, as defined by the number and quality of research publications. Consequently, the salience of research to fiscal fortunes has led to a mounting obsession in academia with both research output and the acquisition of external research funds.

As part of its socialisation process into tertiary education, academic nursing has been similarly been keen to publish credible scientific research. This should have had the effect of raising its status both academically and professionally, while simultaneously laying down the foundations for evidence-based nursing care, yet these outcomes have not materialised. While there has undoubtedly been an increase in the number of nursing research publications, their failure to influence clinical practice in any real way may be attributable to the fact that the nursing process has too often been shaped and moulded to fit the formal scientific paradigm so beloved of academia and health care policists. Not surprisingly, the perceived irrelevance of these studies, focusing as they often do on tortuous reductionist analyses of peripheral nursing issues, described in a new esoteric jargon (Cook, 1991; Warner, 1993), has relegated them to gathering dust on library shelves rather than operating as critical reformers to clinical care procedures. The imposition of the (assumed) high-quality experimental research methodology on the nursing process has undoubtedly rendered a significant corpus of nursing research trivial and clinically inconsequential.

The solutions are obvious if not wholly desirable. The model of nursing care could be modified and reconstructed component by component in order to make it amenable to formal scientific investigation, but this would represent a regressive gesture back to ritualised, task-based care, which has no place within either the new evidence-based health culture or a profession. Alternatively, a more suitable qualitative methodology could be adopted to investigate the nursing process, but this might affect the quality and quantity of research output and hence compromise nursing's status within the academic community. Either way, the relevant knowledge base, so important for evidence-based clinical care, is jeopardised.

One indirect consequence of the implicit propaganda exercise that equates high-quality research with experimental research, is the unambiguous message that it offers the nursing profession: if it wishes to achieve the autonomy, monopolistic knowledge base and status credited with professionalism, nursing must copy medical research in its wholehearted adherence to experimental methods and randomised controlled trials. Nurses are following in the footsteps of doctors yet again, but because this path is an inappropriate one for all the reasons outlined above, their success has been limited, and nurses' servile role relative to the medical profession has been confirmed yet again. What was intended to be a bid for independence and equivalent status within the health care arena has instead been another mortal and retrogressive blow.

THE COST OF THE PROJECT 2000 CHANGES

The shift from apprenticeship training to an academic education was entirely in line with the ingredients of professionalism, but the move to supernumerary status has reduced service contributions over the standard 3-year training period from 60 per cent to 20 per cent. To compensate for this shortfall and maintain an acceptable level of clinical care, there has been an increase in the number of generic health care assistants. Consequently, the profession has lost a considerable amount of territory and numerical power. This position has been made worse by nursing's demand for independent pay bargaining, which, while consistent with professional status, would have resulted in a level of salary expenditure that could not be accommodated within current resources. The 11 per cent reduction in the number of qualified nurses entering the UKCC register and a further expansion in the number of health care assistants have therefore been inevitable consequences (Salter and Snee, 1997).

These educational initiatives, designed to enhance the profession, may instead have weakened its numerical strength. While this, in itself, does not necessarily have a direct effect on evidence-based nursing care, there may instead be an indirect impact. The contracting qualified nursing workforce has experienced not only a decrease in power, but also significantly increased workloads. Hardly surprisingly, the profession is manifesting symptoms of escalating stress and diminishing morale (Tyler and Cushway, 1995). A significant literature exists within psychology suggesting that stress renders the individual or group unreceptive to change, instead adhering to the *status quo* by retreating into well-learned ritualistic behaviours (Menzies, 1970). Applied to nursing, the reduction in collective professional strength that has resulted from the expenditure incurred by the Project 2000 initiative may have generated sufficient threat to retrench care practices in their mechanistic origins while at the same time avoiding research-invoked change.

THE BUREAUCRACY OF THE NHS

The foregoing arguments present only a partial picture, one that attributes blame to the profession collectively. The wider context of the health service within which nursing discharges its services has been a significant contributor to the perseverance of ritualised nursing care. The essential nature of the NHS is bureaucratic, which is typified by Scott (1981):

- an emphasis on universal rules, procedures and regulations
- a strict division of labour
- a formal hierarchical structure
- a clearly articulated line of accountability
- a prevailing concern with conformity and routine, and a lack of interest in individual differences and initiative
- a concern with keeping written records
- a division of the workforce into units, defined by their function.

Thus a bureaucracy is essentially top down, procedural, rule governed and an inhibitor to initiative and autonomy. The NHS reforms of the 1980s were intended to harness the power of the doctors and minimise bureaucratic procedures; however, this has not only been a palpable failure thus far, but also replaced existing structures with the new managerialism. This innovation, while differing from the old bureaucratic structures in numerous respects, has retained many of the characteristics that flawed the previous system and replaced the old sets of procedures with new ones (Davies, 1995). In consequence, the philosophy that views nurses as reflective practitioners, having autonomy, individual accountability and the capacity to modify clinical practice in line with research, is likely to fall at the first hurdle simply because these characteristics offer a fundamental challenge to the bureaucracy within which nurses operate. The very nature of the health service is thus irreconcilable with the independent, innovative practice demanded by its largest workforce.

Other recent reforms have similarly colluded to impede the progress of nursing towards a universal evidence-based care system. Audit, despite its intentions to enhance the quality of care, requires for its success that practitioners adhere to a set of externally determined and monitored clinical procedures. Thus, the decisions regarding acceptable and appropriate care are made not as a result of the nurse reflecting on past and current practices but instead by an external agency. The resulting tension is inevitable. The individual nurse has been officially charged with implementing evidence-based care (UKCC, 1992a, 1992b), yet at the same time clinical practices must be universally prescribed and standardised. As an impediment to reflectivity, innovation and research-informed practice, audit has few parallels.

It would seem that, a decade on, nursing is not much nearer to achieving evidence-based care than it was at the outset, a situation unlikely to alter as long as nurses pursue the holy grail of professionalism and reductionist endeavour. Nor is this stalemate surprising since at every corner nurses find themselves in a dilemma: either existing rituals are retained, with the result that the profession sinks into the mire of unthinking, outmoded practices, or the nurse implements and innovates, thus disrupting the existing social system. Both approaches have a negative pay-off for the individual as well as for the wider organisation, and to this extent, the lack of progress along the road to research-driven clinical care is to be expected. Yet even if there were a paradigm shift and a radical rethink of the end-goals, it is conceivable that ritualistic care would remain embedded within practice.

Such a pessimistic perspective requires explanation. Nursing is the single largest workforce within the NHS, with around 300,000 practitioners on the live register. To imbue this immense cohort with autonomy, independence and an imperative for constantly evolving reflective practice is to challenge the existing power relationships within the health service. The logical end-point of individual authority is a clinical free-for-all, potential anarchy and an irretrievable loss of quality systems and hierarchical structures. The final reality of true professionalism for nursing, with its imperatives for scientifically founded knowledge and independent practice, is in fact incompatible with both the bureaucracy of the NHS and the functioning of its structures. Thus, while government agencies and the professional body openly endorse the value of evidence-based nursing practice, they are simultaneously maintaining the framework that keeps nursing in the barren backwaters of ritual and unthinking habit. There is little doubt that a demoralised, overworked and oppressed workforce is considerably easier to dominate and manage than a large, restless one that is currently baying for full recognition of its unique and complementary contribution to health care. While it is not suggested that this is necessarily a conscious policy, it is nevertheless entirely functional to the management of the system as a whole and the maintenance of the *status quo*.

CONCLUSION

Professionalising nursing has involved numerous policy reforms, which should have both increased workforce autonomy and been instrumental in creating a body of nursing-specific research with the power to inform practice. That clinical practice remains embedded in well-worn ritual may be partly attributable to the unanticipated impact that the major policy changes have had on evidence-based care. Consequently, it is no longer appropriate to hold the individual nurse responsible for persisting traditional clinical practices; instead, the profession and the health service generally must together examine the impact of their own actions and strategies. The promulgation of conflicting messages is well documented as a contributor to psychological turmoil, and as long as nurses are implored to become more research aware and reflective, while simultaneously being constrained in their efforts by various policy initiatives, there will be concomitant confusion and a failure to progress along any useful route. On this basis, then, it is conceivable that evidence-based nursing cannot become a reality until the profession has clarified its essential terms of reference, its corporate values and goals.

The future is not necessarily bleak, however. Nursing has its own invaluable strengths in terms of its practices and protocols; it has no need to refashion itself in the image of academia, science or medicine. To acknowledge this, however, nursing must first be *confident* of its identity and unique role in the system of health care provision. The new face of nursing is still emerging; when the picture is clear, so too will be the nature and role of research in the discharge of care. And if this means that evidence-based clinical practice is temporarily put on hold, then so be it; it is quite probable that its evolution will be an inevitable consequence of professional stability. Perhaps, thus far, too much has been demanded too soon.

REFERENCES

Archer, J. (1992) Gender stereotyping of school subjects. *Psychologist* **5**: 66–9.

Cook, S.H. (1991) Mind the theory/practice gap in nursing. *Journal of Advanced Nursing* **16**: 1462–9.

Davies, C. (1995) *Gender and the Professional Predicament in Nursing*. Buckingham: Open University Press.

Ellis, J., Mulligan, I., Rowe, J. and Sackett, D. (1995) Inpatient general medicine is research based. *Lancet* **346**: 407–10.

Ford, P. and Walsh, M. (1995) *New Rituals for Old*. London: Butterworth Heinemann.

Garmarnikov, E. (1978) Sexual division of labour: the case of nursing. In Kuhn, A. and Wolpe, A.M. (eds) *Feminism and Materialism: Women and Modes of Production*. London: Boston & Henley.

Hicks, C. (1992) Of sex and status: a study of the effects of gender and occupation on nurses' evaluations of nursing research. *Journal of Advanced Nursing* **17**: 1343–9.

Hicks, C. (1995) The shortfall in published research: a study of nurses' research and publication activities. *Journal of Advanced Nursing* **21**: 594–604.

Hicks, C. (1996) Nurse researcher: a study of a contradiction in terms? *Journal of Advanced Nursing* **24**: 357–63.

Hicks, C. (1998a) Barriers to evidence-based care in nursing: historical legacies and conflicting cultures. *Health Services Management Research* **11**: 137–47.

Hicks, C. (1998b) Evidence-based care in nursing: reforms versus research, rhetoric versus reality. *Health Services Management Research* **11**: 246–54.

Hicks, C. and Hennessy, D. (1997) Mixed messages in nursing research: their contribution to the persisting hiatus between evidence and practice. *Journal of Advanced Nursing* **25**: 595–601.

Hicks, C., Hennessy, D., Cooper, J. and Barwell, F. (1996) Investigating attitudes to research in primary health care teams. *Journal of Advanced Nursing* **24**: 1033–41.

Hunt, J.M. (1987) The process of translating research findings into nursing practice. *Journal of Advanced Nursing* **12**: 101–10.

Kaler, S., Levy, D. and Schall, M. (1989) Stereotypes of professional roles. *Image: Journal of Nursing Scholarship* **21**: 83–9.

May, A. (1997) Tried and tested remedies. *Health Service Journal* **107**(5540): 22.

Meerabeau, L. (1992) Tacit nursing knowledge: an untapped resource or a methodological headache? *Journal of Advanced Nursing* **17**: 108–12.

Menzies, I. (1970) *The Functioning of Social Systems as a Defence Against Anxiety*. London: Tavistock Institute.

Peckham, M. (1991) *Research for Health: A Research and Development Strategy for the NHS*. London: HMSO.

Salter, B. and Snee, N. (1997) Power dressing. *Health Services Journal* **107**(5540): 30–1.

Salvage, J. (1985) *The Politics of Nursing*. London: Heinemann.

Scott, W.R. (1981) *Organisations: Rational, Natural and Open Systems*. Englewood Cliffs, NJ: Prentice Hall.

Smith, L. (1994) An analysis and reflection on the quality of nursing research in 1992. *Journal of Advanced Nursing* **19**: 385–93.

Speedy, S. (1991) The contribution of feminist research. In Gray, G. and Pratt, R. (eds) *Towards a Discipline of Nursing*. Melbourne: Churchill Livingstone.

Tyler, P. and Cushway, D. (1995) Stress in nurses: the effects of coping and social support. *Stress Medicine* **11**: 243–52.

UKCC (1992a) *Post Registration Education and Practice*. London: UKCC.

UKCC (1992b) *The Scope of Professional Practice*. London; UKCC.

Waerness, K. (1992) On the rationality of caring. In Showstack Sassoon, A. (ed.) *Women and the State*. London: Routledge.

Walsh, M. and Ford, P. (1992) *Nursing Rituals: Research and Rational Actions*. London: Butterworth Heinemann.

Warner, J. (1993) The empirical new clothes. *Nursing Standard* **7**(31): 47–8.

CHAPTER TWELVE

Implications of policy development for the nursing profession

Peter Spurgeon

Editors' Introduction

This chapter is written from the perspective of someone outside the profession itself. It attempts initially to explore the processes of policy-making, seeing this more as a rather incremental, messy process than as the highly rational and structural procedure it is often assumed to be. Examples are given of policy having a direct impact upon the profession, for example the role of nursing in the purchasing function and in management. The second part of the chapter deals with the need for nurses to influence the development of policy and the need for both greater self-confidence and unity of voice within the nursing body if this is to be achieved successfully.

INTRODUCTION

In trying to understand the implications of health policy development for the nursing profession, there are two distinct and important perspectives to consider. The first may be called reactive in that it is an approach seeking to understand what the consequences for nurses of a particular policy initiative will be. The second perspective is more proactive and attempts to illustrate how nursing as a collective body can influence the shape and implementation of specific policy areas.

The first part of this chapter will be concerned with the reactive aspect by selecting some recent policy developments to illustrate their consequences, both intended and unintended. The latter section will turn to how the profession can (and should) develop stronger processes of influence within policy formulation.

An approach that attempts to describe the consequences of policy developments upon nurses might naturally try to identify specific and precise policy statements on what nurses do or are required to do. This is in practice a rather fruitless and unrewarding approach since relatively few health policies are formulated in this way. Instead, they appear as much more generalised principle statements, and it is much further down the line that consequences appear for one group or another. If this is indeed the case, it may well be because we have tended to misunderstand and therefore misrepresent the concept of policy: 'The very idea of policy implies a degree of orderliness, even consensus; a way forward has been agreed and delineated' (Challis *et al.*, 1994, p. 182). However, this is, by and large, not the case. The argument rests on a conceptualisation of policy as coherent, relatively self-contained and a clear statement of future action. It is a view born of a rational, logical approach to the process of planning and policy formulation. Appealing as this view may be, the reality, especially in the field of social policy, is that it tends to be complex, messy and created within a dynamic environment of competing forces and tensions. Such situations are often described as 'streams of policies' (Webb and Wistow, 1986).

The description of policy-making seems most apt in the context of health care, particularly in understanding implications for the nursing profession. In order to illustrate this situation, one may take as the policy context the set of health care reforms initiated in the UK since 1990, the essence of which has been:

- the separation of the purchasing of health care from its provision, and the use of contracts as a mechanism to relate the two processes
- the creation of NHS Trusts as quasi independent organisations
- the establishment of general practice fundholding (and subsequent developments) with the capacity to hold their own funds and purchase health services on behalf of their patient group.

These developments may be said to have created and to constitute the 'internal market' in health in the UK. Subsequent initiatives, for example evidence-based medicine and the emphasis given to clinical audit and service quality, have added to and reinforced these changes in principle. Perhaps, however, the overall force behind these specific initiatives was that of establishing a financial constraint upon increasing health care costs. Whether expressed through the ideology of market competition, value for money or cost savings, the drive has been to produce a more efficient and more effective health service. An obvious simple consequence of the policy focus upon service quality has been the appointment of senior nurses as quality managers and an increased involvement of nurses in patient satisfaction studies.

However, the majority of policies developed in support of this goal have not contained many direct statements about what nurses should or should not do (*Changing Childbirth*, DOH, 1993, relating to midwives, being perhaps an exception). They have nonetheless had a continued impact upon the nursing profession. In order to illustrate this point, I have selected a number of areas of policy from these 'streams of policies' and attempt to show how they affect nursing.

EXAMPLES OF POLICY DEVELOPMENTS AND THEIR IMPLICATIONS

Nurses in purchasing

It is probably fair to suggest that purchasing as a new concept in the health service was not at the outset particularly well understood. Expertise has slowly grown, and more mature purchasing approaches can be seen in the 3–5 year developmental agreements and in the greater collaboration between purchasers and providers in dealing with some of the issues of the reconfiguration of services and cost pressure. An obvious imbalance in the purchasing process was in terms of access to medical/clinical input, purchasing authorities being dependent upon in-house public health doctors, perhaps some locality general practitioner representatives and maybe independent clinicians outside their own population area. In contrast, providers have had access to the full range of clinicians and other professionals. The new Labour government's emphasis upon collaboration between health organisations may well encourage a greater participation and sharing of this clinical expertise.

Nurses were often absent from the purchasing process or, where they existed, their role was unclear. This seems particularly odd when one considers that 80 per cent of direct patient care is delivered by nurses, midwives and health visitors. Their close contact with patients would suggest a valuable input into contract specification. However, the lack of involvement of nurses suggests that they did not figure prominently in the initial policy discussions of how purchasing should be accomplished.

A study by the NHS Executive (1993) confirmed that the nursing contribution to purchasing was limited and that it seemed to be largely directed at a quality assurance aspect. The report did, however, usefully identify some of the key areas of potential contribution from nurses:

- challenging clinical practice as a credible group respected by other staff and patients
- challenging the basis of prices from their awareness of the calculation of nursing costs
- evaluating alternatives in the way in which services are provided
- interpreting users' needs.

A more recent study (Pursey and Brocklehurst, 1996) suggests that nurses in health authorities frequently contribute in other functional areas (contracting, organisational development and community relations), and their nursing background is seen as bringing added value but not as being essential. In their work with a particular health authority, the authors suggest that one way forward would be to identify a lead nurse in each of the authority's main purchasing areas (primary care, priority services, acute services and continuing care). This would go some way to bridging the gap as nursing practice issues can be underrepresented in contract discussions. It does of course also require a recognition on the part of the providers as well as the direct involvement of nurses in contract negotiations – again, something that is not always common practice.

Purchasing therefore seems to be an area in which the content and requirements of contracts have major implications for nurses but is a process to which they have not yet made a full contribution. One observes here a typical reactive policy issue whereby the formulation of the purchasing process has tended to marginalise nursing involvement while, through the setting and specification of contracts, having a significant impact upon the work of nurses. Indeed, studies of morale, motivation and stress in nursing staff suggest that the impact is even more negative, nurses feeling alienated from decisions concerning the nature of services and frustrated by not being able to deliver care to the level and standards they would wish because of a combination of workload, resource constraints and inflexible contracts. It is argued by Littlejohns *et al.* (1996) that multiprofessional advisory groups are essential if locality-based purchasing is in future to be established as a representative and effective process. Nurses must be full partners in these groupings.

It is interesting to note that the Labour government's White Paper on the future of the NHS places nurses at the forefront of commissioning within the community and/or primary care groups.

Nurses and doctors – role boundaries

A quite specific national policy has been to limit the hours worked by junior doctors. However, the time reduction has not been linked to additional resources, and the work remaining must therefore be undertaken either by the consultant grade or via an expansion of the nursing role. The latter has been an option followed in a number of areas. Many in the nursing profession welcome this long-awaited opportunity, believing that the potential for releasing nurses' skills has been stifled by the defensiveness of the medical hierarchy. Others, however, are more cautious, being aware of both the general increase in nursing workload and the issue of legal responsibility involved in any transfer of tasks.

A study by Dowding *et al.* (1996) examined the implementation of four new nurse practitioner roles. Although they were largely successful and exciting, and welcomed by the majority, the study suggested a lack of clarity surrounding the accountability attached to the new posts. While not wishing to dampen the entrepreneurial spirit in taking on such new roles, the authors advocate a close involvement of the nurses themselves and the professional bodies in agreeing and setting new guidelines on accountability in new areas of practice.

There are, however, a number of areas of successful practice in this sphere. One such area involves prescribing by nurses. Following an audit of the delay in patients receiving their required drugs, the Royal Alexandra Hospital for Sick Children in Brighton introduced limited nurse prescribing. The success of the scheme resulted in (Barnes and Fox, 1995):

- an improved preparation of children for painful procedures and appropriate responses to each child's needs
- junior doctors being relieved of some onerous prescribing duties
- an expansion of the nursing role, with both quality and financial implications.

Similar developments are occurring in primary care, with nurse practitioners expanding their roles, most typically into areas such as women's health, common and minor illnesses, and special clinics (asthma and diabetes). All these of course require general practitioner collaboration but again perhaps point the way for a more effective utilisation of nursing skills and indeed improved patient services.

It is worth noting, however, some of the tensions and perhaps inherent conflict in some of these policies. For example, *Changing Childbirth* (DOH, 1993) as a policy document places the mother at the centre of maternity care and emphasises a greater choice in the pattern of care, as well as offering greater continuity from the professional staff providing the care. The latter aspect translates for the most part into midwifery-led care. It seems to allow midwives to operate as autonomous professionals, much as they have advocated. However, the emphasis on continuity requires that midwives offer intrapartum care as well as ante- and postnatal care. This is of course challenging not only in terms of skills and responsibility, but also in terms of the time demands upon the individual midwife. The unpredictability of individual mothers' birth times tends to mean that midwives have to be increasingly on call. It is somewhat ironic that as one national policy strives to reduce working hours for junior doctors and seeks to allow general practitioners to opt out of 24 hour cover, midwives are at the same time being encouraged (directed) in the opposite direction. It would thus seem that the process of the substitution of one professional by another, although offering opportunity, must be examined closely in terms of respecting the needs of other individuals and groups. It is also an example of 'streams of policies', in which the underlying coherence is not always immediately obvious.

Nursing and research

Over the past 5 years, the place of research in the health service has become more and more important. Evidence-based medicine and the need to rationalise services by concentrating on only that which is effective has necessitated this shift to a research-based culture. This is, however, a rather centrally driven process with a national R&D directorate. It is also a rather medically dominated process, the randomised controlled trial being seen as the gold standard for research and by some as the only proper form of research. So where does nursing research, with its frequently qualitative emphasis, fit into this scenario?

Hicks (1995) also comments upon this apparent mismatch when discussing the relative lack of published research from nurses despite the national emphasis on a research-based health service. She highlights the perception of research as essentially quantitative and large scale as being a contributing factor. It is also apparent that there is a lack of confidence within the nursing profession concerning the appropriateness of researching the softer, more qualitative issues so often implicit in the more holistic concept of health care embodied in the nursing process. There is an awkward tension here, the research culture pressing for a more and more scientific basis to health care delivery, often leading to a dissection of the care process and the more integrative orientation of nursing education. Furthermore, one might search in vain for evidence that nurses, under increasing pressure of workload, will be given more free time to undertake research. Again, it feels like a 'left hand versus right hand' policy formulation.

There is perhaps a suggestion inherent in the struggle to develop an evidence base for nursing of the continuing obstacles to the profession becoming a more active influence upon the policy development process. A number of independent but interrelated factors conspire to inhibit more active involvement.

These forces include:

- an unhelpful historical stereotype of nursing as reactive, passive and compliant; the recent emphasis upon the reflective practitioner of course offers a counter to this view, but to the extent that it is still held, it nevertheless acts as a block to active engagement and collaboration in constructing new policies
- a persistent and continuing gender-specific identity, the associated feminine values not being perceived as valuable for leading radical change
- a spate and speed of reforms, policy changes and initiatives that has made it difficult for nurses to be involved in shaping the policies or indeed for allowing time for particular changes to embed themselves within the professional culture.

Nurse management

As a final example, we might consider the process of nurse management. This in some ways represents a policy predating the 1990 UK reforms. The origins of reform in the UK system can be seen in the mid-1980s with the implementation of the Griffiths report (DHSS, 1983) recommendations: that the NHS was poorly managed and that there was therefore a need to import management practices and managers from the private sector into general management posts. Thus, the concept of general management was introduced into the NHS.

Part of the thinking behind this initiative was a belief that the medical profession, still operating within an administered health service, was overly dominant and therefore not accountable to anyone. The merits of the approach are not really appropriate to debate here. The point can, however, be made that the nursing profession fared badly within this process, very few general managers being appointed from a nursing background. This may of course have been owing in part to the sense that general managers were there to 'control' doctors, thus making it difficult to appoint nurses because of historical relationships. Conversely, it raises the question of why experienced nurse managers were not deemed to be appropriate for appointment as general managers.

Edwards and Roemer (1996) perhaps offer some clue to why this might have been the case. In a study of four teaching hospitals, they report that nurse managers' perceptions of their own skills and the importance they attached to certain areas of management gave rise to a positive focus on the operational tasks of management. Where managers felt less well equipped was in terms of managing the external relationships of their organisations. In times of major change, the absence of such skills may be seen as being crucial to general management. Perhaps a lesson to be drawn here is that the profession must attempt to blend internally focused management competence with a more strategic, external approach encompassing a wider environment of influences.

The negative consequence of the new managerialism for the nursing profession is acutely observed and described by Davies (1995). She relates the difficulties once again to the gender base of nursing, suggesting that nursing management tasks are seen as feminine, that is, dealing with staff issues, and are therefore regarded as rather internally orientated management processes. As a reaction to this view and culture, nurses themselves internalise their focus, defend their nursing empire and therefore further isolate themselves from issues such as service development and, in the context of this chapter, policy development.

INFLUENCING POLICY

This selective analysis has identified areas in which policy initiatives, although not specifically targeted at particular groups, have significant consequences for the work and functioning of the nursing profession. We have seen this in terms of new roles, new demands and workload. The challenge as presented here is generally one of nurses 'doing more' but thus also of the opportunity to develop. In addition, the potential threats must be recognised. For example, the drive to reduce costs could also mean that trained nurses might be replaced by more generic health workers able to undertake some less technical nursing tasks. This thus represents a situation in which nursing is responding to policy, sometimes benefiting but at others experiencing greater pressure. This may at times produce defensive reactions, but at best it can be rather passive. It is important to turn to how nurses can become more proactive and influence the shape of future policy.

Laschinger and Havens (1996) suggest that the proper empowerment of nurses is an important component of this. In a study assessing professionals' views of their own roles, these authors found that where empowerment offered real autonomy and control over the content of their work, much greater satisfaction and effectiveness were perceived. One conclusion, then, is that the profession must continue to ensure that status equal to that of all other care professions is attained and therefore to increase discretion and direction over work tasks. This enhanced ownership is more difficult than it would appear at first glance. It requires clarity regarding the care or essence of nursing and a willingness to recognise when some tasks and activities are more dubious. Thus, an initial requirement for a greater involvement in policy is that the profession must be clear and confident about its contribution, and see how this extends to external as well as internal influence.

This is of course easier said than done, in part because of an inherent problem of the size and diversity of the profession. The perception that the professional bodies have been concerned to defend territory and perhaps focus upon internal disputes may be unfair, but it certainly exists. Can the nursing profession in its widest definition unite and speak with one voice? Its diversity and diffusion is both a strength and weakness. It is, however, the latter that represents a difficulty in offering a clear and powerful view as policy issues are debated.

Part of this growth may be supported by the clinical supervision initiative in the UK. This process, offering peer-based supervision, is aimed at supporting individual nurses as well as improving overall organisational systems and ultimately improving patient care. Although in its early stages, it offers a further opportunity for developing skills and confidence in the participants, as well as identifying critical skills within the profession.

In order for nursing to acquire a more influential proactive role, a number of important transitions may be needed. It appears that the profession must be very clear about its knowledge, skills and potential contributions – as we have seen in purchasing, management and so on. But competence must be allied to confidence and an awareness of how such knowledge can contribute to the policy formulation process. Nursing still feels 'operational'; indeed, it is to the 'hands-on' nurse that the public conveys its affection. Very few nurses are active in the policy arena. This is partly historical, and partly the result of misconceptions about the value of nurses to policy development both from within and outside the profession.

The growth of academic nursing departments is both an index of the situation and an opportunity for the future. Why has nursing taken so long to integrate with the academic community? Why is the involvement in nursing research so small relative to the total number of staff employed? Overcoming this position is part of the requirement to move nursing into strategic arenas and policy areas. Nursing policy units might be a positive organisational development. At the same time, this is not an academic problem. It is vital too that, in order to be significant in the policy area, nursing must develop a clearer and stronger sense of unity about what it wishes to say, and this will also require the development of effective mechanisms for collecting the views of nurses at the grass-roots level.

Mulhall (1996) believes that nursing has a great opportunity to make use of the increased emphasis upon epidemiology and evidence-based patterns of health care and to be at the forefront of patient-based care systems. She believes that some new skills in epidemiology and research will need to be acquired but that nurses' traditional concern with quality of care gives them a head start in assessing the outcomes of care processes.

Change is clearly continuing for the health service and for the nursing profession, but opportunities for growth also exist.

REFERENCES

Barnes, J. and Fox, D. (1995) *Nurse Prescribing on Children's Wards*. VFM Update. Leeds: NHS Executive.

Challis, L., Fuller, S., Henwood, M. *et al.* (1994) Investigating policy coordination: issues and hypotheses. In McKevitt, D. and Lawton, A. (eds) *Public Sector Management: Theory, Critique and Practice*. London: Sage.

Davies, C. (1995) *Gender and the Professional Predicament in Nursing*. Buckingham: Open University Press.

Department of Health (1993) *Report of Expert Maternity Group (Changing Childbirth)*. London: DoH.

Department of Health and Social Security (1983) NHS Management Inquiry. The Griffiths Report. London: DHSS.

Dowling, S., Martin, R. and Skidmor, P. (1996) Nurses taking on junior doctor's work: a confusion of accountability. *British Medical Journal* **312**: 1211–14.

Edwards, P.A. and Roemer, L. (1996) Are nurse managers ready for the current challenges of healthcare. *Journal of Nursing Administration* **29**(9): 11–17.

Hicks, C.M. (1995) The shortfall in published research: a study of nurses' research and publication activities, *Journal of Advanced Nursing* **21**: 594–604.

Laschinger, H.K. and Havens, D.S. (1996) Staff nurse work empowerment and perceived control over nursing practice. *Journal of Nursing Administration* **29**(9): 27–35.

Littlejohns, P., Dumelow, C. and Griffith, S. (1996) Knowledge based commissioning: can a national clinical effectiveness policy be compatible with seeking local professional advice? *Journal of Health Service Research Policy* **1**: 28–34.

Mulhall, A. (1996) *Epidemiology, Nursing and Healthcare*. Basingstoke: Macmillan.

NHS Executive (1993) *Building a Stronger Team: The Nursing Contribution to Purchasing*. Leeds: DoH.

Pursey, A. and Brocklehurst, N. (1996) Developing the Nursing Contribution to Purchasing. Unpublished report. West Midlands Regional Health Authority.

Webb, A.L. and Wistow, G. (1986) *Planning, Need and Scarcity: Essays on the Personal Social Service*. London: Allen & Unwin.

CHAPTER THIRTEEN

From profession to commodity: the case of community nursing

Nicola Walsh and Pippa Gough

Editors' Introduction

*This is an insightful chapter commenting on the impact of policy develop-
ments in primary health care and their influence on community nursing.
A historical outline describes the rise of medical dominance in the
primary care field, with the transformation of community nursing into a
commodity that meets the requirements of contracts. The deleterious
effect that policies can have on the nursing profession becomes painfully
obvious in this chapter. The incremental development of these policies
may have undermined the influencing ability of nurses over time, or
perhaps nurses were busy focusing on patient care, as they should, while
not also keeping their eyes on what was coming over the hill. Whatever
nurses could have done, it would not have been strong enough to counteract the powerful voices of the doctors and managers.*

INTRODUCTION

This chapter charts the slow but discernible shift in the status of
community nursing from that of a loose grouping of diverse professionals with their own professional priorities and aspirations to a
commodity shaped and driven by the contract culture of the market.
This development has mirrored the political drive to create a 'primary
care-led NHS' – a move that has marginalised nursing and given scant
attention to its contribution to the attainment of primary health care
in the broadest sense. Recent policy initiatives have sought in minor
ways to address this erosion of professional integrity, but the power to

negotiate and set contracts, and within these to dictate the nature and direction of nursing practice, has to a greater extent been left in the hands of the medics and managers.

The focus of this chapter is the current structure of our health services within the community rather than the quality or nature of care being delivered, although oblique reference may be made to this at times.

Community nursing seems to have been largely overlooked by those developing the policy and practice of what is now known as 'a primary care-led NHS'. It is still being treated as an appendage, yet it is a vital part of primary health care in the UK. Policy-makers, managers, nurses and other professionals need to look carefully at the nature of the service and recognise the importance of some of the more visible aspects of nursing work. Professional roles are being redefined and the relationship between the public (state) and the private (market) is being rapidly altered.

Just like other professional groups, community nurses have accommodated internal (service-specific factors) and external (political, social and economic factors) change in the past. What, then, has been the impact of the internal market upon nurses working within the community? This chapter assesses the implications for community nursing of this new relationship between state/market and public/private, and suggests that the very nature of and belief in community nursing as a professional entity in its own right, with its own priorities and direction, have been stripped away. Today, it is more easily recognisable as a commodity that is shaped by the demands of the market and whose existence is dependent upon inclusion in the fine print of contract specifications, usually drawn up by medical staff and managers. So how did this happen, and what does this mean for the future shape and content of community nursing?

The chapter attempts to provide some of the answers, and to do this it is divided into four sections. The first section explores, in some detail, the history of the NHS from the perspective of the development of primary health care. These key developments of the past provide clear portents of the current commodification of community nursing and the rise of medical dominance in the primary health care field. The next section considers the impact of the NHS and Community Care Act 1990 upon nurses in particular and other professional groups in general. The third section explores some of the potential implications of recent White Papers, especially *Choice and Opportunity* (DoH, 1996a) and *Delivering the Future* (DoH, 1996b), as well as the NHS (Primary Care) Act 1997, which received royal assent in March 1997. The final section concludes with some suggestions on the nature of primary health care nursing in the future. For the purpose of this chapter, the term 'community nursing' is used to describe the work of all nurses working in patients' homes, as well as those involved in preventive, screening and health promotion work in local primary health care settings. This includes district nurses, health visitors, practice nurses and community-based specialist nurses.

PRE-1990

Until the 1950s, district nursing was dominated by voluntary associations, while health visiting was always accepted as part of state health service provision. Even where voluntary workers were involved, health visiting activities were supervised, directed and often largely financed by local authorities (the state). Health visitors were viewed as a vital extension of the Medical Officers of Health in their surveillance of local populations. However, district nursing, like midwifery, had an uncertain margin between the practitioner and the handywoman. These differences continued to shape the two areas of work through the two World Wars and into the NHS.

District nursing remained marginal to the state, although it became identified increasingly as a branch of nursing. Health visiting, on the other hand, grew more important to the state as it became more involved in the problems of maternity and child welfare. As the number of health visitors increased, so too did the scope of their work. Some doctors, however, did not accept their expanded role/responsibilities; for example, their involvement in antenatal care was seen as a threat by some general practitioners, although others welcomed the extra referrals from this aspect of health visiting intervention. Health visiting was also not fully accepted by the nursing profession – indeed, this 'separatism' was mutual, some health visitors fighting explicitly for the recognition of health visiting as a profession in its own right. Unlike district nursing, therefore, it remained marginal to the larger nursing profession.

Although maternity services continued to be a policy priority after the Second World War, health visiting seems to have lost ground in two directions. It failed to resist the encroachment of social work into its traditional domain of child welfare, and it failed to colonise the new territories of work in the community with the old, the chronically sick and the mentally ill. Although health visitors have, at various times, been used to provide services to one or other of these client groups since 1945, in none of them have they actually secured a long-term position as the dominant service provider.

While health visiting drifted in a policy vacuum during the post-war period, it is arguable that district nursing fared rather better. The NHS Act of 1946 obliged local authorities to provide a free home nursing service, so district nursing came to be subsidised by the state. Embodied in the 1946 NHS Act was also a clause enabling local authorities to set up health centres in which general practioners could rent surgeries to dispense their medical services, alongside domiciliary nursing and midwifery, health visitors, social workers and other services for which the local authority itself was responsible. In the event, little use was made of this statutory provision in the two decades that followed the Second World War, and the different professional groups continued to operate from separate premises (Webster, 1993)

With the establishment of the NHS in 1948, the state became the primary payer and provider of health care (Leathard, 1990). As a consequence, health care professionals played a key role in the allocation of state resources. It was the 'era of the professional' (Alazewski, 1995). Professionals had the confidence of the general public, and members of the public could directly access a number of different health care professionals – a situation now inhibited and constrained by the prevailing 'contract culture' that requires a much tighter gatekeeping of services. There was also a political consensus about the role of the state in health care provision. General practitioners enjoyed a form of delegated discretion in their role as 'gate-keeper' to secondary care, while district nurses and health visitors enjoyed 'the less rule-bound' environment of the community, working autonomously and often in isolated settings, drawing upon the medical practitioner and other therapists only as and when necessary.

With the publication of the Family Doctor's Charter in 1965 (Taylor and Bloor, 1994), a variety of measures were introduced that provided favourable conditions for the development of primary health care. The notion of primary health care teams (PHCTs) was introduced, aimed at bringing family doctors together with health visitors, district nurses and other staff employed by local authorities in health clinics. As a result, health centres were established at a hectic pace between 1966 (25) and 1976 (731) in an attempt to forge closer links between general practice and community health services (Webster, 1993). This provided opportunities to co-ordinate and integrate curative, preventive and rehabilitative care.

It is interesting to note that the introduction of the Charter in 1965 was prompted by a growing belief that the failure of community-based staff to work together effectively was leading to a greater pressure for hospital admission (Taylor and Bloor, 1994). In order to facilitate this process still further, the 1974 NHS reorganisation initiated the transfer of community health services from the local authority to hospital control. However, far from prompting the development of enhanced team work, it is arguable that this 'closer working' served only to allow the medical dominance of community nursing to assert itself even more. Twenty-one years after this concept of the PHCT had first been articulated formally as a policy goal, the Cumberlege report (DoH,1986) was to pronounce it a failure of massive proportions on precisely these grounds. The report developed a helpful critique at the failure of the PHCT and set out numerous recommendations to ameliorate future working.

The workload of community nurses began to change and increase as their work became more directed by requests from family doctors to carry out delegated 'general medical services'. As a consequence, district nurses increasingly delegated 'non-nursing duties' to assistants working in the NHS and to home helps from social services. Meanwhile, health visitors developed a philosophy that almost denied their clinical nursing role in favour of their health promotion, community development and social care roles. When their 'hands-on' nursing skills were called upon, they tended to refer their patients to another part of the service (Robinson, 1985). Thus, within the parameters of growing medical influence, new 'care' boundaries were also being set by nurses themselves. This was further strengthened with the implementation of the Mayston committee recommendations (DHSS, 1969), a community version of the Salmon report (MoH, 1966). A new breed of nurse administrator was introduced, these people effectively removing themselves from direct patient care, and in one fell swoop the practice-based, clinically expert and experienced senior community nurse began to disappear overnight. The notion of expertise and expert practice in relation to *caring* and *care* interventions (the work of nurses) was thus rapidly deconstructed, a move from which community nursing has struggled to recover ever since. Government policies, albeit unintentionally, were redefining the boundaries of nursing care. As a consequence, the confidence of nurses and the expert contribution of community nursing, over and above those activities delegated by the general practitioners, began to be subtly eroded, and the nature of the nursing care within the community became narrower and defined more tightly by the medical model.

In 1979, a Royal Commission report stated:

that there was considerable scope for expanding the roles and responsibilities of health visitors and district nurses. (p. 79, para 7.26)

This report recognised the:

> increasingly important role for community nurses not just in the treatment room but in screening procedures, health education and preventative programmes, as a point of first contact particularly for the young and the elderly. (p. 79, para 7.26)

So, as was the case in other countries at this time (Alma Ata Declaration, WHO, 1978) the government began to acknowledge the enormous potential of the nurse's role within the development of true primary health care. Pragmatism, however, rather than ideology was the heart of this renewed investment in nursing ability; part of the rationale for expanding the role of community nurses arose from the fact that more and more people were being discharged back into the community at a much higher level of dependency. It was financially and politically expedient.

The case for extending the frontiers of community nursing was reinforced by the publication of the Cumberlege report on community nursing services (DoH, 1986). This was part of the Green Paper on primary health care services issued by the government in April 1986. In the report, Cumberlege recommends the introduction of the nurse practitioner, extended powers of prescription for a limited number of items, and the setting up of neighbourhood nursing services to draw nurse managers back into clinical practice and reverse the effect of the Mayston report. Cumberlege's report also suggested that there should be locally negotiated, written agreements concerning objectives for the primary health care team. This proposal attracted more opposition than many of the others since it symbolised the fact that nurses in the community would be making an agreement as equal partners with general practitioners on what services should be delivered, how they would be delivered and by whom.

In its initial response to the Cumberlege report, the medical profession was rather hostile to the ideas of an expanded role for nursing, and, as in the mid-1970s, the government were reluctant to act as it would involve 'tampering with the territory of the medical profession'. Yet, paradoxically, many doctors were at the same time arguing for an extension to the ancillary payments scheme that would allow them to employ more nurses to relieve them of a whole range of tasks of the preventive kind identified by Cumberlege. With the election of a Conservative government in 1979, 'committed to reducing public expenditure, rolling back the state, and challenging the public sector and professional monopolies' (Flynn, 1992, p. 7), the autonomy of the professional began to be questioned, and, with the introduction of general management in the mid-1980s (DHSS, 1983), the 'frontier of control' shifted from professionals to managers. No longer were decisions made by a group of professionals through consensus: it was the health service manager who took overall responsibility. To some extent, the impact of these changes was more cultural than structural (Oakley and Greaves, 1995). Managers became increasingly involved in decisions about health care as 'choices' taken at a managerial level began to determine the parameters in which care and treatment decisions were taken at an individual level.

Within hospitals, managerial influence grew as information technology improved and managers were able to assess the workload and resource usage of nurses and doctors, and thus the costs of treatment. In the community, this 'commodification' of care was far more difficult. IT systems were often not available, and the nature of the care was not easily translated into discrete, quantifiable episodes. The fact that primary care centred on people and relationships rather than bricks and mortar also influenced the nature of managerial control. Unlike the bureaucracies and hierarchies of a hospital, community health services relied far more on a collegiate structure. They were 'network' organisations with less hierarchical relationships between colleagues and more developed, collaborative interagency relationships. It took at least another 10 years before managerial influence, to the level of that in hospitals, began to be extended into primary care.

The government's active stance towards 'primary care' – a phrase denuded of the word 'health', indicating the increasingly reductionist approach that was taken later – began with the publication of the White Paper *Promoting Better Health* (DoH, 1987). This essentially represented the government's terms for negotiation with the profession and signalled an increasing emphasis on the 'new managerialism'. It displayed a shift away from respecting professional autonomy, giving greater recognition to the 'choice' of the consumer. The same themes of better value for money through stronger management, which characterised policy in the hospital sector, were also reflected. This report highlighted the government's aims in primary care, including that of giving higher priority to health promotion and illness prevention (Ranade, 1994).

It also demonstrated for the first time the placing of the lead for primary (health) care with the general medical practitioner and general practice. Thereafter, the term 'primary health care', and more recently 'primary care', was to become increasingly interchangeable and finally synonymous with general practice and the role of general medical practitioners. This is explicit in the new NHS (Primary Care)

Bill (1996), wherein the entire concept of primary care becomes fully interchangeable with the notion of 'personal medical services'. For community nursing, this has proved to be very damaging.

Not surprisingly, the government and the medical profession failed to reach agreement on translating the primary health care philosophy that emerged in the 1980s into a mutually acceptable system of incentives built into general practitioner contracts. Instead, the government insisted on a rigid system of incentives, such as the health promotion banding payments and medical audit – failure to agree resulted in the unilateral imposition of the 1990 general practitioner contract. In the wake of these policy developments the work of many community nurses, which centred on a more holistic and expanded notion of primary health care, became increasingly invisible. The further away from, and more out of step with, general medical practice and the work of the general practitioner this type of nursing activity appeared to be, and the less under its control, so its importance and legitimacy decreased proportionately. Public health work, community development activities and broad health promotion strategies were no longer commodities regarded as essential for the new primary care/general practice.

Instead, those facets of nursing placed *within* general practice began to flourish. General practitioners were given incentives under the 1990 contract to employ practice nurses to carry out 'general medical services' that could be delegated. Practice nurses, focused on individualistic intervention and confined to the surgery (and thus not infringing the private space of the home), became the nursing *Zeitgeist* and reflected the overall demise of health care as state intervention. In their ascendancy, practice nurses grew from 9,000 in number in 1986 to 17,000 by 1995 (Atkins and Lunt, 1993). Other community nurses, such as health visitors, born of welfarism and the notion of the public state were less defined and therefore could not compete, instead becoming easy prey for those managers seeking cost-efficiencies.

THE NHS AND COMMUNITY CARE ACT 1990

This Act introduced radical reforms to the way in which the health service in the UK was organised and financed. From April 1991, district health authorities became purchasers of health care on behalf of their resident populations and began to relinquish managerial responsibility for their local hospital and community units. The provider units began to apply for self-governing status, and a contractual relationship was introduced between the health authority and the Trust. Providers no longer had a guaranteed budget to pay for the service they delivered; instead, they had to engage in a competitive process of winning contracts in order to secure an income. Health authorities were responsible for assessing the health care needs of their resident populations and for commissioning health services that best met those needs within the resources allocated to them. A centralised administrative structure was replaced by a more pluralistic set of arrangements in which competition, as well as management, determined how health care services were to be developed (Ham, 1994).

Health authorities were not the only purchasers of health care: general practitioners could also opt to receive a budget from which they could purchase a limited range of services and goods for patients registered with them. Initially, the general practitioner fundholding scheme was restricted to practices with a list size of 9,000 or more, and the budget covered some hospital services, drugs and practice staff. Each year, the list of services and goods widened, and in April 1993, community nursing services were added to the list (via contracts with community Trusts), reflecting the organisation of primary care services around a practice-centred system of management. General practitioners began to specify the nature and volume of community services they required and, in some cases, the actual preferred individuals who would perform these tasks. These new arrangements replaced the previous 'attached' model, whereby nurses employed by the local community Trusts worked with certain general practitioners and were based at the same health centre or clinic. As a consequence, relationships of authority and responsibility between and within the different professional groups were radically altered. In some cases, district nurses and health visitors became practice employees, and historical loyalties to their own professional group weakened as they developed an increased commitment to the practice.

The introduction of the internal market has also altered public access to broader primary health care services. General practitioner approval is increasingly required before community nursing services are made available. The role and value of certain nursing activities and disciplines are also increasingly being questioned by general practitioners and managers as the caring activities are defined and costed for contract negotiation and specification. This often reduces nursing to a mere list of disaggregated tasks. This is particularly so in relation to the public health role of health visitors – which in the notorious 'red book' is allowed to account for 10 per cent of their time. As public health/community development work is often a philosophical approach as much as a set of activities, contracting on this basis has rapidly become meaningless.

Part of the problem may lie in a lack of understanding of the role. This could be because the health visitor's direct interaction with general practitioners is often limited, frequently amounting to a shared child health clinic. In contrast, district nurses tend to have daily inter- action with general practitioners, if only to get prescriptions signed, opportunities for developing informal relationships and a clearer understanding of roles thus being enhanced. Moreover, district nursing is largely concerned with secondary intervention and care, which equates more easily with the general practitioner's role. Health visiting, on the other hand, remains a more alien concept. Questions by doctors and health service managers on the value of health visitors may lie in the fact that underlying principles of health visiting – identi- fying health needs and enabling people to take control of their health – rest awkwardly in the current structure of the NHS, focused increas- ingly as it is on secondary care interventions. Responding to *health* need, as opposed to the need for *health care*, is arguably no longer seen as either feasible or desirable within the current NHS.

Health visiting derived its legitimisation from a growing sense of responsibility by the state for, and a public interest in, the early detec- tion and remedy of incipient cases of disease or handicap. It is essen- tially concerned with surveillance of the private space of people's lives. In today's ideological climate, such surveillance is generally seen as undesirable, although the state still demands it vigorously in particular instances, for example cases of child abuse. Since 1990, there has been a discernible shift in the nature of health visitors' work from routine home visits to clinic-based work in order to accommodate these changes and become a more legitimate and marketable commodity. In addition, clinic work by health visitors is an attractive commodity for general practitioner practices, helping as it does to fulfil vital aspects of the general practitioner's contract.

Other changes introduced through the NHS and Community Care Act 1990 included the transformation of family practitioner commit- tees to family health service authorities. This introduced a different culture into the organisation and management of general practi- tioners. The Act also gave local authorities the ability to purchase welfare services from the independent sector. The role of the local authorities changed from being direct service providers to 'enablers' (Ham, 1994). As with health care, contracts were to be used to specify the type of service to be provided, the method of payment and the monitoring arrangements. District nurses in particular were affected by these changes as some 'nursing' activities were increasingly provided by personnel working in the independent or local authority sector. Boundaries were formally redefined between health and social, formal and informal, care. As a consequence, the role of the state in the provision of care has altered considerably. The nature of caring and what is purchased legitimately as 'health care' has also been narrower. Many dimensions of nursing are now only finding expression outside the NHS – or not at all. This is particularly so in relation to public health work (as discussed above), the therapeutic aspects of mental health nursing – now so often reduced to interventions aimed at custody and control – and some dimensions of palliative care and complementary therapies.

Within the contract culture, a greater fragmentation of tasks and functions within both nursing and new professional groups is becoming apparent. One effect of such divisions of labour is the potential loss of continuity and coherence of care. A particular patient may be handed from one professional to another as problems emerge; the home of a family needing help or support can sometimes seem like a busy hospital ward without the security of that environment. In fact, despite the ethos underpinning the drive towards care in the community, individuals now run the risk of being institutionalised in their own homes or dropping through the net altogether. The introduction of a market-based system of health care was framed by the political values of the time: greater economic efficiency, individual choice and personal responsibility. In the mid-1990s, such values are being replaced with notions of 'community responsibility', a shift reflected in recent government policies that place a greater emphasis on devolved decision-making structures and local public involvement.

THE PRIMARY CARE-LED NHS

Throughout 1995, the government focused its attention on the development of primary care by conducting a 'listening exercise' with appropriate professional groups. The outcome of this exercise has been a spate of White Papers, the most important of which is *Choice and Opportunity. Primary Care: The Future* (DoH, 1996a), which has initiated the new NHS (Primary Care) Bill. The essential proposal behind this White Paper and the attendant legislative changes is to enhance the delivery of primary (health) care by removing the structures that have been prohibiting greater flexibility in the provision of what are known as 'personal medical services', that is, that job for which general practitioners have traditionally been contracted. Although these 'personal medical services' have, over time, come to embrace a diversity of different services – some routinely provided by nurses, in fact – it is alarming that a major policy document purporting to concern primary *health* care is in fact focused exclusively on the delivery of *medical* care. For nurses, the implications of this terminological and conceptual sleight of hand are worrying. In the future, will mainstream nursing in primary care be that which most closely mirrors medical practice? And if this is the case, whither those aspects of nursing concerned with the principles of broader health promotion, the search for health need and the optimisation of individual and community health status? What is clear is that, where community nursing is concerned with the delivery of 'medical care', the White Paper appears to allow this type of nursing to begin to assert itself as an entity rather than a commodity appearing on someone else's contract. From this perspective, the White Paper provides opportunities for nurses to establish a more equal relationship with general practitioners. With legislative change, nurses will formally be able to be taken on as equal partners within a practice. The number of nurse practitioners will increase, so the number of nurses directly engaged in the critical tasks of the diagnosis and prescription of care will rise. Much of this 'new role' will be facilitated by the full implementation of nurse prescribing. For the rest of community nursing and its broader dimensions, the status of commodity remains, and with that, the dominance of the contract and the loss of professional self-direction will prevail.

The reforms laid out in the White Paper will formalise the purchaser/provider split in primary care, and many of the new arrangements envisaged are dependent upon a greater use of contracting. Local contracts between health authorities and 'new' primary care providers may be introduced in order to deliver that which has previously been provided wholly by general practitioners. Within this, the notion of subcontracting becomes increasingly more likely as new primary care organisations located around general practice begin to subcontract for the non-medical aspects of their activities. As the contract culture grows and develops in complexity and sophistication, the danger is that the focus will be on contracts rather than on the process of care. Thus, as in secondary care, managers – albeit in some cases a general practitioner turned manager – will control decisions. This raises many questions about the role and responsibilities of nurses in these new primary care organisations. A greater use of contracts will require greater accountability, but what currency will be used in contracts and, more importantly, how will these contracts be monitored? For community nursing, the answer to these questions may point to a bleak future.

Local contracts have the potential to increase flexibility, but if this approach is left to develop without state intervention, it could result in new private conglomerates controlling large portions of primary health care. This is particularly the case in disease management packages where there is pharmaceutical company involvement. Current proposals suggest that the health authorities will provide public funds, and regulate activities, through contracts. Should partnerships evolve between the commissioners of primary health care and the commercial sector, however, there is obviously a danger that the regulatory role of the state may be reduced or shared between other interests.

CONCLUSION

Hunter (1995) has argued that the NHS has always been a marketplace. Before 1991, the market was a political and sociological one in which the currency was the shifting power relations between various stakeholders. Since 1991, the 'notion of the market has become narrower and more restricted with economic considerations uppermost' (Hunter, 1995 p. 23).

Saltman and Von Otter (1995 p. 248) have suggested that the 'current mixed stage of development of planned markets reflects uncertainty as to exactly where an appropriate social and economic balance lies'. The balance of social and economic responsibility ultimately reflects the values of society at large. If the focus continues to be on economic rather than social policy, there are dangers that the regulatory and funding role of state in health care provisions may well diminish altogether. Nurses in the future may well be working in quasi-independent organisations that are partly controlled and funded by commercial bodies, thus altering the nature of public care.

Greater local diversity in both the purchasing and the provision of primary health care services may mean that, in the future, the universal availability of services to all members of society is uncertain. The process of contracting may also lead to a greater duplication of some services and gaps in others unless health authorities undertake to co-ordinate and regulate provision. It is possible that the proposals in the White Paper *Choice and Opportunity* (DoH, 1996a) could replace the individual set of relationships between doctor and patient, and nurse and patient, with an organisational relationship. This may mean the ultimate commodification of both medicine and nursing. However, given the whiphand of medicine in the current 'primary care-led NHS' (which has not been addressed by the new Primary Care Bill), it is unlikely that primary *medical* care will be reconstructed as a commodity in the same way as is happening to nursing. Nursing, on the other hand, is offered no such freedom and will continue to have to fight to control its own professional destiny.

Since this chapter was written, we have seen two key policy changes introduced by the Labour government that may influence the role of nurses within primary health care.

First, we have seen the establishment of primary care groups. Although general practitioners will be in the majority, each primary care group will have one or two nurses on its board. With 480 primary care groups being set up across England, this means that about 1,000 nurses will be involved in commissioning who did not previously take part. However, the real challenge will be for the nurses involved in these groups to commission for *health* and not just for personal medical services.

The second key policy change introduced by the Labour government that could affect developments in community nursing is the Green Paper *Our Healthier Nation* (DoH, 1998). This paper acknowledges the glaring evidence that health depends on social, economic and environmental policies as well as on individual lifestyles and health services. The government wishes to see tackled not just the causes of disease, but also the causes of those causes, for example poverty, unemployment and all other features of the social and physical environment that converge to undermine health. Health visitors could play an important role in addressing this huge agenda: they have some crucial skills that could be used by primary care groups to identify the health needs of their populations.

However, they, like other professionals, will have limited success unless they build alliances with other professional groups and local bodies. In the future, health visitors will need to move towards the surveillance of public issues that affect health and be less focused on the surveillance of people's private lives. Such new roles will obviously need to be recognised by the general practitioners – otherwise we may see this group of nurses being marginalised even further.

REFERENCES

Alazweski, A. (1995) 'Restructuring health and welfare professions in the UK: the impact of internal markets on the medical, nursing and social work professions in Johnson, T., Larkin, G. and Saks, M. (eds) *Health Professions and the State in Europe.* London: Routledge.

Atkins, K. and Lunt, N. (1993) *Nurses Count: A National Census of Practice Nurses.* SPRU: University of York.

Department of Health (1986) *Neighbourhood Nursing, A Focus for Care* (Cumberlege Report). London: HMSO.

Department of Health (1987) *Promoting Better Health*, Cm 249. London: HMSO.

Department of Health (1996a) *Choice and Opportunity. Primary Care: The Future*, Cm 3390. London: HMSO.

Department of Health (1996b) *Primary Care: Delivering the Future*, Cm 3512. London: HMSO.

Department of Health (1998) *Our Healthier Nation: A Contract for Health.* London: HMSO.

Department of Health and Social Security (1969) Report of the Working Party on Management Structure in the Local Authority Nursing Service (*The Mayston Report*). London: HMSO.

Department of Health and Social Security (1983) NHS Management Inquiry Report (*Griffiths Report*). London: DHSS.

Flynn, R. (1992) *Structure of Control in Health Management.* London: Routledge.

Ham, C. (1994) *Management and Competition in the NHS.* Oxford: Radcliffe Medical Press.

Hunter, D. (1995) Dealers must listen to healers, *Health Service Journal* 22: 23.

Leathard, A. (1990) *Health Care Provision: Past, Present and Future.* London: Chapman & Hall.

Ministry of Health. Scottish Home and Health Department (1966) Report of the Committee on Senior Nursing Staff Structure, Chairman Brian Salmon, Ministry of Health. London: HMSO.

Oakley, P. and Greaves, E. (1995) Restructuring: decentralisation, *Health Service Journal*, (9 Feb): 30–1.

Ranade, W. (1994) *A Future for the NHS?* London: Longman.

Robinson, J. (1985) Health visiting and health. In White R (ed.) *Political Issues in Nursing: Past, Present and Future*, Vol. 1. Chichester: John Wiley & Sons.

Royal Commission on the National Health Service (1979), Cm 7615. London: HMSO.

Saltman, R. and Von Otter, C. (1995) *Implementing Planned Markets in Health Care.* Milton Keynes: Open University Press.

Taylor, D. and Bloor, K. (1994) *Health Care, Health Promotion and the Future General Practice.* Nuffield Provincial Hospitals Trust, RSM.

Webster, C. (1993) 'Mobilisation for total welfare, 1948 to 1974' in Webster, C. (ed.) *Caring for Health: History and Diversity.* Milton Keynes, Open University Press.

World Health Organisation (1978) Alma Ata 1978: Primary Health Care. Geneva: WHO.

CHAPTER FOURTEEN

Influencing and implementing policy reforms – a practical perspective

Sylvia Fry

Editors' Introduction

This is a very practical and personal account of one director of nursing. She describes using all available opportunities to ensure that local knowledge and expertise were made available to influence and shape local policies for the implementation of national policies. She concentrates on the health and social care interface and describes her role as a nurse executive influencing her own corporate agenda. The importance of understanding the bigger picture and applying local knowledge to the development of appropriate local implementation policies is illuminated in this chapter. The interaction between other policies, for example those on education, housing and the environment, with health are emphasised. Managing the nursing involvement in many different policy agendas is another key feature.

INTRODUCTION

Executive directors of NHS Trusts are responsible for ensuring the delivery of a high-quality service, viable in business and financial terms and able to identify and develop potential new business. It is therefore apparent that directors must be fully aware of national developments, using all opportunities to ensure that local knowledge and expertise is made available to influence and shape such policies. The nurse director must balance this corporate role with the professional role of leading the nursing function within the Trust.

In this chapter, we will consider some of the complex changes that have occurred within health care over the past 5 years and the way in which nursing developments within the Trust have not only been responsive to these changes, but are also able to influence future local and national policy.

SETTING THE SCENE

Southern Birmingham Community Health NHS Trust provides a wide range of care to a population of some 420,000 people. Its services include a dental teaching hospital; the largest outpatient genitourinary medicine service in the West Midlands; specialist intensive rehabilitation services, including access to communication and technology; inpatient care for young physically disabled people; a day centre for head injury rehabilitation; peripatetic services for people with brain injury; inpatient, respite and day hospital care for elderly people; and the traditional community services. In 1996/97, the Trust had an income in excess of £56 million and employed over 2,100 staff. Of these, almost 900 worked within the nursing service.

Since our formation, from six different units, in 1991, we have been working within the 'Trinity of Aims', which can be identified in all major policy statements and initiatives within health care. These are:

- improving the quality of patient and client care
- achieving a greater responsiveness to the needs of individuals
- better value for money.

A Vision for the Future (NHSME, 1993a) highlighted that the success of current developmental policies such as the *Health of the Nation* (DoH, 1992), *Caring for People* (DoH, 1989) and the *Patient's Charter*, (DoH, 1991) together with others such as *New World, New Opportunities* (NHSME, 1993b), *Research for Health* (DoH, 1993) and *Working in Partnership: A Collaborative Approach to Care* (DoH, 1994) depended significantly on the contribution of skilled and committed nurses, health visitors and midwives.

It is therefore apparent that, for any Trust, a nursing workforce ready and able to take on these challenges is vital for the successful development of its business. As the Nurse Director, I have the task of ensuring that nursing developments are appropriate to the corporate direction of the Trust, as well as having wide-ranging operational management responsibilities.

INFLUENCING THE CORPORATE AGENDA

Influencing strategic change

While the advent of Trusts has brought about an increased emphasis on strategic provider planning, a down-side was the recognition that there was no 'right of access' to the decision-making process within the purchaser arena. At a stroke, one felt excluded from many of the traditional settings for service planning, for example health care planning teams. The internal market meant that colleagues of long standing were seen as competitors rather than comrades. These problems were probably made more acute in Birmingham because of the fact that the social services department was concurrently undergoing its own organisational change. There was thus a high need for identifying other means of influencing health care policy.

In terms of the health–social care interface, implementing the major policy directives such as *Caring for People* (DoH, 1989), meant that there was a high need for multiagency working task groups. Within these groups was a recognition that new methods of mutual working and influencing would be required. One such group formed following public health work on the impact that social changes were having on children's services. Birmingham now has a family support strategy, accepted by both the city council and the health authority, with input from every statutory agency in the city. This group will soon be able to be disbanded, the ongoing work returning to within the joint planning arena. With the maturing of both purchaser and provider organisations has come a return to a more 'partnership' approach to care planning, although it is clear that the use of more short-term informal working groups will continue.

In terms of health care, this came mainly through general management and its responsibility for contract negotiation. In a sustained period of reducing financial investment in community services, it was clear that nursing advice was at a premium if cuts were to be made with the least possible effect on the quality of patient care.

For the Trust to continue to succeed, there had to be a recognition that the only constant feature was that of change! The change agenda included that of developing staff, especially nurses, who are the largest single group of staff, not only for the 'here and now', but also for beyond the usual strategic period. The agenda for the Nurse Director was to concentrate on the visionary state and scenario-planning, ensuring that staff were flexible and professional enough to deliver care in any organisational structure in the future. We have to develop a workforce that, while being big enough to be compared to an oil-tanker that requires 3 miles to stop, has the capacity to behave like a canoe, able to change direction rapidly and smoothly with the touch of a paddle.

Developing strategic responses

Perhaps the unique challenge of working within primary and community services is the complexity of working on so many boundaries. We work at the interface of:

- health and social services
- health and education
- health and adult recreational and community services
- health and independent providers of care
- health and the voluntary sector
- health and environmental services.

The relationship between poverty and health needs is now well established, so education, housing and environmental policy all have a major impact on both health care delivery and health care planning. Policy changes in any of these interrelated areas may have long-term implications for future developments in community nursing. In terms of business planning, they may bring threats to our business, but they could also bring opportunities for the expansion of services or for improving quality.

The Carers (Recognition and Services) Act 1995 places a duty on social services departments to assess the abilities of a carer who is providing substantial amounts of care to someone on a regular basis. This duty extends to their taking this assessment into account when deciding what services to provide to the person to whom care is being given. What, then, are the implications for the Trust, as a health care provider, of this Act? At first sight, there are very few implications, until it is put alongside the *Patient's Charter* (DoH, 1991) and the increasing expectations of the population for the delivery of health services that are appropriate to their individual needs.

Patients' complaints have been given a high priority within the *Patient's Charter.* I would contend that this has led to a much-improved approach to these complaints. Indeed, within my own Trust, all compliments and complaints are considered by a Trust board committee. As a member of that committee, I carefully examine all complaints that have nursing implications, partly to consider whether trends or common issues can be identified. What is apparent is that, even if all clinical care has been appropriate, if patients have themselves been kept informed and carers have been given information, carers may still find it difficult to accept the changing circumstances in which they find themselves – or the person for whom they are caring. Nurses are good at considering the implication of such changing circumstances on their patient and the immediate environment and can facilitate such recognition. For the past 6 years, I have been privileged to be an invited member of the Birmingham Carers Panel and have seen a clear development of carers recognising that they are essential components in the delivery of care. They have challenged the traditional community nursing prioritisation of caring first for patients who depend totally on statutory care, followed by patients who have their own carers. Rightly, they have identified that the cost saving to the NHS is high and thus argue logically that carers should have the highest priority.

How, then, should we, as a community Trust, respond to the needs of the carer?

- What service development is needed to support carers, in terms of equipment, training in their tasks or respite care, to name but a few of their needs?
- Should we be continuing to develop partnership working with voluntary agencies, thereby being able to offer a lower cost option to health authorities?
- With which local groups should the Trust be developing such partnerships?
- How will we ensure that quality of care is maintained when we are offering expertise within a package of care being mainly provided by other staff, and what accountability for nursing standards do we have in such a situation?
- Are we sure that NHS responsibilities and developments are consistent with the spirit and the framework of the Act?
- Is this consistent with our core business? And if so, can we afford not to recognise the implications of the interlinked but very separate policies?

I would suggest that such issues are clearly within the remit of the Nurse Director and, indeed, could not be effectively considered without a clear view of the implications for nursing as a whole.

Developing the Trust nursing strategy

Workforce planning, including skill mix exercises, is an essential prerequisite for working in this developmental way. Link-workers, advocates and interpreters are all essential components of both nursing teams and the wider primary health care team. Policies such as *The New Deal* (NHSME, 1991) have also impacted on nursing development. More and more, our nurses are active in defining and setting standards of care within multidisciplinary and multiagency frameworks. It is therefore essential that the roles of individual team members are clearly understood by all and that role changes between professional participants are introduced by mutual agreement. To facilitate this, a nursing strategy has been adopted within the Trust. This has identified 10 key characteristics of nursing practice from national policies and guidelines:

- accountability
- clinical skills
- the use of research
- teamwork
- innovation
- health promotion
- staff development
- resource management
- quality of care
- the management of change.

These are alongside eight key features needed to maintain a learning organisation:

- an articulated policy
- effective communication
- the involvement of stakeholders
- performance review
- clinical supervision
- providing a learning workplace
- reflective practice
- the translation of rhetoric into practice.

Only by providing an environment that enables clinical practice to develop and flourish will an organisation be able to deliver on the requirements of national policy.

Improving the clinical environment

With the emerging emphasis on a service based around general practice populations, it became clear that service delivery changes would have a major impact on the estate requirement of the Trust. We operate from over 30 bases, with a correspondingly high level of capital charges. Many of these premises had major problems in backlog maintenance. Apart from inner city partnership-funded health centres, there had been very little investment in community premises over the previous 20 years or so. Some premises were converted council houses, with major security problems because of their isolation and having only two or three staff based within them.

The biggest stumbling block to developing this approach has been the private finance initiative. Most of our schemes are relatively small in capital development terms. The redevelopment and refurbishment of centres may cost between £300,000 and £600,000; a new build will be in the order of £1 million. Local requirements are often highly specific to that area and to the local community. Our general practice colleagues, being used to 'Red Book' arrangements, are often incredulous at the process that the Trust has to undergo. These inbuilt delays are contrary to the need for responsive and flexible approaches. Perhaps the most difficult task of all is when, as in one building, we are jointly working with other organisations and the success of our scheme also depends upon developing a scheme that fits the philosophies of those other organisations.

It was a clear responsibility of the Nurse Director and local managers to identify the type of clinical accommodation that would be needed in the future. We recognised that our core business was in the delivery of care rather than in real estate. With a great deal of co-operation from the then family health services authority, individual general practitioners and staff, a strategy has been developed that will enable a much-reduced number of buildings to remain, complementing local practice accommodation and situated in major areas of high public health need. Such buildings had to assume the type of nursing care that would be delivered for at least the next decade and the consequential accommodation needs.

This scenario building of future service delivery then had to be translated into bricks and mortar.

THE NURSING AGENDA

Responding to a primary care-led NHS

The development of general practitioner fundholding in Birmingham was slow. Indeed, in 1993/94, the Trust was working with only five fundholding practices. Community services for the other 103 practices were delivered within one contract with South Birmingham Health Authority. These fundholders were located in practices that were to some extent already working within the concept of primary health care teams. They therefore had higher activity levels than many other practices. Ironically, just at a time when indications were that the health authority would be looking to purchase care with regard to health needs rather than on historical patterns, the ability to reprovide on a more equitable basis was removed.

Despite the administrative complexity, it became rapidly apparent that the purchasing of health care was carried out in a much more realistic way when a practice was deciding the requirements for its patients than within a large amorphous contract. It was also apparent that many practices wanted a higher involvement in how nursing care was to be delivered. Most problematic was the indication that practices preferred a discrete nursing team. While this was possible for large practices, it was clear that as more smaller fundholder practices came on stream, it would become more and more difficult. Indeed, with the number of staff employed, it would be impossible. This issue was made more acute by the fact that, having implemented a skill mix exercise in district nursing the previous year, we had reorganised into larger nursing teams, increasing the middle-grade staffing numbers and reducing the number of team leaders.

The decision was taken that we should anticipate all general practitioners becoming fundholders, that nursing teams had to be capable of delivering care within the philosophy of individual practices and that this would mean differing skills and training needs being met according to practice needs. Thus, while recognising the universality of NHS care, we were also recognising that, in business terms, it was the general practitioner rather than the patient who was our customer. Nursing teams were reorganised around groups of practices. In the outer city, this required relatively little change as group practices were common and clear practice boundaries were in operation. Much more difficult were the inner city areas, with a high number of single-handed general practitioners whose patients were frequently scattered over a very wide area. We recognised that there would be an added (and unfounded) cost in terms of higher mileage and a reduced amount of time available for patient contact. Concurrently, the health authority was looking for increased activity as a measure of cost-efficiency.

Our predictions that these changes would bring about more effective liaison between community and practice staff were correct:

- Nursing staff now undertake joint training
- Projects are underway in implementing models of joint assessment for the cost-effective delivery of nursing care
- Practice protocols are in operation in a number of clinical areas.

We have, however, also been the victims of our own success. We have seen an overall increase in general practitioner referrals to community nursing by 25 per cent (in one instance by 100 per cent). A similar increase has occurred in the provision of home equipment. Staff are undertaking 30,000 more home visits per year, only slightly compensated for by the fact that more appropriate teamworking has reduced the input into surgery clinics by some 7,000 contacts. This, together with Birmingham's traffic calming measures, has led to an increase in annual mileage of over 38,000 miles. In reality, this additional mileage equates to the loss of 1.8 'G' grade nurses. We are also seeing an increasing number of high-dependency patients, our hospital colleagues routinely discharging patients requiring ongoing care in terms of such techniques as enteral feeding.

The newly merged Birmingham Health Authority of 1995 recognised the strength of the fundholding model but also identified that, in order for the 'primary care-led' NHS to develop, there was a need for a much higher involvement of all general practitioners in commissioning services. A purchasing model emerged of grouping likeminded practices into primary care commissioning groups. These were composed of both fundholding and non-fundholding practices. Three of the four pilots that were set up had community services provided by the Trust. Other fundholders preferred to remain as 'stand-alone' practices and still others were part of a Multifund organisation. The result of this development is that, in 1997/98, we hold nursing contracts with:

- 28 fundholding practices within South Birmingham
- 9 fundholders in adjacent areas
- 6 fundholders who are also members of primary care commissioning groups

- 9 practices who are members of primary care commissioning groups
- 1 health authority, on behalf of the remaining 56 general practices.

We believe that the larger primary care commissioning groups will enable a better utilisation of nursing staff, not only in terms of care continuity for patients and more cost-effective visiting patterns, but also in recognising and developing individual staff members' special expertise and professional interest.

There are so far no primary care commissioning groups served by the Trust that are based in inner city areas. The recognition of the differing styles of service delivery to defined client groups is of high importance. For example, Birmingham has a small but growing Yemeni community, residing across a wide geographical area but who register mainly with a general practitioner well versed in their culture and religion. Such individual practice needs may be better served by a higher emphasis on group health needs rather than geographical population needs.

Similarly, there is a range of specialist nurses who may be caring for a defined population such as travellers and homeless families. Other nurse specialists are employed for patients with specific disease conditions such as stoma care; they, again, because of their number, do not readily fit into a primary care team. *Choice and Opportunity* (DoH, 1996a) provides the ideal vehicle for developing the innovative integration of such services with primary care commissioning groups.

Implementing nursing care developments

In financial terms, Birmingham Health Authority was currently deemed to be 3.5 per cent (£15 million) over budget. Indeed, it was anticipated that 1997/98 would see a reduction of £4.9 million. This obviously brought much additional strain on services that had year on year been producing higher levels of activity. However, as the Secretary of State wrote in the White Paper, *A Service with Ambitions* (DoH, 1996b, p. 5):

> the human and financial resources available to the NHS are necessarily limited. It is the task of everybody in the NHS to ensure that patients secure the maximum possible benefit from them. The search for better and more efficient ways to meet the needs of patients must be relentless.

It is therefore important to consider whether nursing can show the appropriate clinical developments at all levels and within all disciplines that have enabled policy directives to be fulfilled. It is also appropriate that we should review whether the continuation of these developments will assist in reaching the key objectives set out in this policy document.

'A well-informed public'

There is a welcome recognition within the document of the need rapidly to improve the information infrastructure. Just as importantly, there is a recognition of the need to improve public information on services, treatment options and outcomes. In the Trust, we recognised that for some communities, especially those from different cultures, additional assistance and education needed to be provided before information channels such as telephone helplines and written information could be appropriately accessed and used. Within the health visiting service, we had already developed the use of community link-workers. These posts, relating to specific health visitor caseloads, took health advisory programmes to minority ethnic groups. In addition to providing information, this was an ideal method of identifying the health issues of most concern to such groups. From such work, a group of isolated women with high health needs was identified. A 3-year project was set up, not for the provision of information but for the provision of an advocate for women. As a result of this programme, the women set up their own health group, and identified their own information needs so successfully that the health promotion department was then able to obtain funding to develop posters and supporting material for *Health of the Nation* (DoH, 1992) topics geared specifically to their needs.

The school health service was, several years ago, refocused from being a primarily generic screening and surveillance service to one that was also geared to identifying specific areas of health needs within defined school populations. This led to the recognition that many teenagers were baby-sitting when they had little or no knowledge of the responsibilities that such duties entailed. Some youngsters were concerned about this and felt that first aid training would be beneficial. The school nurses recognised that a more structured response was required. A 'baby-sitting course' and supporting manual have been produced. The emphasis of this educational course is obviously one of providing basic child care information. Its underlying theme is to ensure that these teenagers are aware of the wider health issues that parenting brings (such as passive smoking) as well as of how they can best access child care services. The approach of listening to the school-child and developing a response to these vocalised needs also facilitates the disclosure of hidden concerns. In one school, this was the identification of a number of young people who were taking on major caring responsibilities. Following this, the school and our carers support initiative have set up a young carers group through which emotional and practical support can be given. It is fair to say that most of the group members were unaware of the facilities that were available to them from the health and local authority services.

'A seamless service'

In an attempt to overcome traditional organisational boundaries and clarify roles and responsibilities, Birmingham nurse managers and social services managers jointly agreed an approach termed *The Wavy Line* (Birmingham City Council Social Services Department *et al.*, 1994). The document attempted to identify when it was appropriate for the different services to undertake care, while recognising that each situation was unique and the boundaries of care therefore needed to be flexible to those needs. This was a useful tool, and local joint training on its implementation also greatly assisted the process of multiagency working. It was apparent that, with the implementation of the Community Care Act, there was a need to further develop joint working.

There also seemed to be little provision for nurses to become care managers even when there was a high level of health-related care need. Our response was that, following discussion and negotiation with the social services, we altered the role of the elderly care visitor to one of a community-care co-ordinator. These post-holders undertook care management training with their social work colleagues and were then based for half of their working week in the local social services offices. They participate fully in the 'access' function of the social services team and take on care management in which complex health care issues are apparent. Thus, when continuing care legislation needed to be implemented, we were in the fortunate position of having staff well prepared to take on this role. Our next task is to determine how these posts can better relate to primary care teams without disrupting the social services link. Similar posts are now in operation within the major acute Trusts with whom we work.

Nowhere is this seamless approach to care more apparent than in the provision of 24-hour intensive nursing packages to severely disabled people. Early this year saw the return to our community of a small boy with tetraplegia. After a road traffic accident, this child had required 2 years inpatient care at a national specialist hospital in another part of the country. Throughout that time, his mother had stayed with him at the hospital and his sisters had been cared for by grandparents while his father maintained the family home in Birmingham. His return home required the co-operation of every public service, as well as a housing association to provide custom-built accommodation for the child and our nursing staff. The clinical care package has involved the setting of protocols with our local children's hospital in order that intensive care facilities are available for emergency situations. Protocols have also needed to be developed with the ambulance service and the specialist hospital for when they would expect him to be returned to their care. Our care is provided not only within the home environment, but also at school. Indeed, as he became of school age during his hospital stay, this schooling commenced before his discharge, and nursing staff and educational staff travelled to the hospital to undertake training and orientation. Of course, the care package must include the psychological impact that the situation has had on the whole family. The provision of such care identifies that high technical nursing skills can be provided within community settings. We have needed to identify the competences and skills required to deliver such care in order to provide safe, high-quality care at the most economic cost.

'Knowledge-based decision-making'

In common with most Trusts, we are committed to developing clinical audit and ensuring that the clinical effectiveness of service provision is identified. Interestingly, we are beginning to see that patient surveys in preventive health care provision can be used as an indicator of effectiveness. For example, in a survey of health visiting client satisfaction, we identified that, after health visiting intervention:

- 34 per cent of the clients changed the care of their baby
- 4 per cent changed their own health care activities
- 11 per cent changed their home environment.

In another project aimed at increasing the uptake of immunisation and cervical cytology, a baseline questionnaire found that although 70 per cent of the women had heard of cervical cytology, 50 per cent were not aware of the need for 3-yearly testing. At the conclusion of the project, a questionnaire found that 80 per cent of the women felt better informed, 50 per cent said that they intended to attend for return appointments and 60 per cent said that they would encourage other women to attend.

More in-depth research has been undertaken using the Edinburgh scoring system as an indicator of postnatal depression (see Elliot, 1996). Following the progress of those clients involved over a period of 12 months, it can be seen that there is a positive relationship between health visiting intervention and a reduced score. These results were presented to the general practices whose patients were involved in the study, and discussions are now well in hand concerning the implications for the team and the respective roles of the team members in the management of postnatal depression. The approach has also been developed further in one inner city area to meet the specific needs of women from minority ethnic populations.

'A highly trained and skilled workforce'

One of the issues facing community Trusts is the lead time that it takes for staff to become appropriately qualified for this work. It is obvious, therefore, that high-quality community experience for students is an essential component of the nursing services.

It is also important that we are able to influence educational establishments in their selection process. For some time, we have been involved with a local university in this way for the selection of degree nursing students. What is apparent is that we are not seeing applications from minority ethnic students appropriate to the population mix. Our development of training for interpreters and link-workers has led us to consider whether alternative career entry pathways could be developed. With the support of the NHSME (1993b), we are on the point of being able to have such a training course accredited as an entry qualification at diploma/degree level in nursing. This will complement and supplement the accredited courses that we have already developed in an inner city area for training local people to provide lay health advice.

'A responsive service'

A common thread throughout all such developments is the recognition that the needs of communities vary. In order to be sensitive to patients' needs and wishes, services must be able to be provided in a sensitive and flexible way.

The start of such recognition is the development of caseload profiles. However, if developed as a stand-alone tool for nursing, they lose much of their potential. Such profiles must be seen as an integral part of the practice profile, which in turn relates to the wider population profile of a prescribed area. At that point, profiles become effective planning tools for commissioning as well as assisting in individual and team caseload management and sensitive service delivery.

Within the Trust, we have for some years used first parent visiting as a means of targeting health visitor resources. With caseload profiling came the recognition that this was not the delivery method of choice in all areas. We have thus seen two additional models being used. In one locality where there is a high population of young, non-English speaking parents, one project is working with first-time parents using a totally user-focused rather than professionally focused approach. A steering group of young mothers is directly influencing the way in which the project evolves. A very different style of working is taking place in a fundholding practice situated in an outer city area with high deprivation levels. Here, we employ a nursery nurse working under the direction of the health visitor to undertake a specific programme of practical support to the parents, including skill-building in child stimulation and parenting skills. This work directly links into a nearby community facility where play workers are involved. Thus, there is a natural progression from a health service to other local services. Both these projects have the same aim but, to be responsive to local needs, use very different approaches.

THE WAY AHEAD

The DoH White Paper (1996b) states that:

> Our ambition is for a high-quality, integrated health service which is organised and run around the health needs of individual patients, rather than the convenience of the system or institution. An NHS which, where appropriate, brings services to people, balancing, for each individual, the desire to provide care at home or in the local community with the need to provide care which is safe, high-quality and cost-effective.

Such an ambition will continue to challenge every aspect of nursing practice in general and community care in particular. Perhaps the biggest challenge for nurses at Trust level is to ensure that examples of high-quality, cost-effective care are appropriately resourced and integrated into mainstream service delivery.

REFERENCES

Birmingham City Council Social Services Department and Birmingham Health Authorities and Trusts (1994) *The Wavy Line: Home Care and Community Nursing Working Together.* Birmingham: Birmingham City Council.

Birmingham Health Authority, *Draft Purchasing Plan* 1997/98. Birmingham: Birmingham Health Authority.

Department of Health (1989) *Caring for People: Community Care in the Next Decade and Beyond*, Cm 849. London: HMSO.

Department of Health (1991) *The Patient's Charter.* London: HMSO.

Department of Health (1992) *The Health of the Nation: A Strategy for Health in England*, Cm 1986. London: HMSO.

Department of Health (1993) *Research for Health*. London: DoH.

Department of Health (1994) *Working in Partnership: A Collaborative Approach to Care: Report of the Mental Health Nursing Review Team* (Chair: Professor T. Butterworth). London: HMSO.

Department of Health (1996a) *Choice and Opportunity*. London: Stationery Office.

Department of Health (1996b) *A Service with Ambitions*. London: Stationery Office.

Elliot, S. (1996) *Postnatal Depression: Focus on a Neglected Issue*. London: HVA.

NHS Management Executive (1991) *Junior Doctors: The New Deal*. London: Stationery Office.

NHS Management Executive (1993a) *A Vision for the Future: The Nursing, Midwifery and Health Visiting Contribution to Health and Health Care*. Heywood: DoH.

NHS Management Executive (1993b) *New World, New Opportunities: Nursing in Primary Health Care*. Heywood: DoH.

CHAPTER FIFTEEN

A final postscript

Peter Spurgeon and Deborah Hennessey

The process of health system reform is taking place in many countries throughout the world, and many new models are evolving. Political and financial turbulence, advances in medical technology and changing expectations are all part of the background to these changes. They are also the reasons why nurses, as the most numerous professional grouping within health care, must be influential in shaping the outcome of these various forces. This text has tried to illustrate the many settings (practice, education and research) where this can, and should, take place. Examples have been given of where the influence of nursing has been evident in policy formulation and reformulation. At the same time, failure to influence policy has been discussed and the sense of marginalisation highlighted.

There are many strands to this process. Key aspects will include establishing an evidence base for nursing practice, embedding research, both qualitative and quantitative, in the culture of the nursing profession, and creating a strong, clear, confident and as far as possible unified view of what the profession wants and in which direction it is seeking to move. Policy developments in the context of global information access will be increasingly international, although different constraints and opportunities will of course present themselves within different health contexts. For example, in the UK, the potential impact of nurses with epidemiological skills within the commissioning role of the new primary care groups is considerable.

In order to have the impact they should have, nurses will need to equip themselves with the necessary skills, expertise and confidence to operate as equal status professionals within the primary care team. The whole thrust of a primary care-based service, alongside the pressure on available doctor input and the advanced nurse practitioner role, provides tremendous opportunities for the nursing body.

This text has attempted to demonstrate, encourage and cajole nursing to take up this challenge. Perhaps the overriding requirement if we are to move beyond an enthusiastic subgroup to involving the whole body of the profession is to develop a clear vision of future direction, to communicate this clearly and to establish the relevant forums for the message, and thereby its influence, to be heard.

Page numbers printed in *italic* refer to tables; a letter n following a page number denotes a note number on that page.